T0302216

Resilient Health Care

Resilient Health Care

Volume 6

Muddling Through with Purpose

Edited by
Jeffrey Braithwaite, Erik Hollnagel,
Garth Hunte

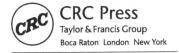

CRC Press

Taylor & Francis Group
Boca Raton London New York

CRC Press is an imprint of the
Taylor & Francis Group, an **informa** business

First edition published 2021
by CRC Press
6000 Broken Sound Parkway NW, Suite 300, Boca Raton, FL 33487-2742

and by CRC Press
2 Park Square, Milton Park, Abingdon, Oxon, OX14 4RN

Library of Congress Cataloging-in-Publication Data
Names: Braithwaite, Jeffrey, 1954- editor. | Hollnagel, Erik, 1941- editor.
| Hunte, Garth S., editor.
Title: Muddling through with purpose / edited by Jeffrey Braithwaite, Erik
Hollnagel, Garth Hunte.
Description: First edition. | Boca Raton, FL : CRC Press, 2021. | Series:
Resilient health care ; volume 6 | Includes bibliographical references
and index.
Identifiers: LCCN 2020046852 (print) | LCCN 2020046853 (ebook) | ISBN
9780367558031
(hardback) | ISBN 9781003095224 (ebook)
Subjects: LCSH: Health facilities--Personnel management. | Health services
administration. | Organizational resilience.
Classification: LCC RA971.35 .M83 2021 (print) | LCC RA971.35 (ebook)
| DDC 362.1068/3--dc23
LC record available at https://lccn.loc.gov/2020046852
LC ebook record available at https://lccn.loc.gov/2020046853

ISBN: 978-0-367-55803-1 (hbk)
ISBN: 978-0-367-55804-8 (pbk)
ISBN: 978-1-003-09522-4 (ebk)

Typeset in Times
by Spi Global, India

Contents

Part I   Openings

Part II   Case Studies of Muddling

Part III   The Functional Resonance Analysis Method (FRAM) as a Gateway into Muddling with a Purpose

Part IV   Muddling with Application: In and Around Hospitals

Part V Closure

Preface

The world of health care is changing. Among other things, there are pressures on budgets, new models of care, resource-constraints, creeping bureaucratic requirements and shifting demographics. There are also new technologies, drugs and techniques; new patient populations with greater and more complex needs than ever before; and many competing demands on clinicians providing frontline care. Indeed, the challenges to providing high-quality care are considerable, and often daunting. It is easy to criticise; however, among all this, stakeholders get by, and perform effectively across-the-board, from frontline through to governments. Clinicians mostly offer good, safe care. Managers and leaders endeavour to create organisations in which services are well-received and supported by the community. Many policymakers and politicians try to build environments in which people can do well, responding to the needs of their population.

It is convenient to assume that when the health system performs successfully, the reason is that it's because the guidelines are being closely followed, policy is being faithfully carried out, rules are being consistently adhered to and norms specified by administrative decision-makers are the dominant way work is undertaken. We have come to label this Work-as-Imagined.

In truth, work was never this rational; it was never able to be specified so perfectly, or prescribed so clearly – not even in simpler times, and especially not today. Instead, work is carried out in flexible and infinitely varied ways, adjusting to circumstances, exigencies and demands that change from minute-to-minute in busy environments, grounded in the knowledge and expertise of the professionals. People are not robot-like automatons but agents with agency. They make compromises, take shortcuts, trade-off efficiency and thoroughness and navigate complexity, to the best of their ability.

In short, providers muddle through with purpose, built on expertise and wisdom. And that is what this book is all about – the capacities of people in health care to do what they can to get things done regardless of the conditions under which they labour.

I warmly invite you to read on, if you are interested in safer, higher quality care, as explicated by some of the best thinkers and writers on the ideas of resilient health care. Over the last few years many of these ideas have borne fruit, exposing how care is actually delivered rather than how some people imagine it is delivered.

It's hard to believe, in fact, that this is Volume 6 in the Resilient Health Care series. Building on the other five, this volume offers an intriguing perspective on the muddling paradigm. I have therefore one piece of advice to my colleagues: read on – you will benefit tremendously from the wit, wisdom, analysis and perspectives on muddling through as shown here.

Wendy Nicklin, RN, BN, MSc(A), CHE, FACHE, FISQua, ICD.D, President, International Society for Quality in Health Care, 2017-2020

Acknowledgements

Our sincere thanks to all our authors who amidst the global pandemic of Covid-19 and the demands it has placed on their lives have been able to contribute deeply insightful chapters exemplifying with conceptual clarity the idea of what it means to muddle through with purpose. It is testament to their commitment to patients and providers everywhere.

We also thank the editorial team at the Australian Institute of Health Innovation, Sydney, Australia for their assistance in the creation of this sixth installment of the Resilient Health Care series. Dr Wendy James copy edited some of the chapters. Our research assistant team of Kelly Nguyen and Kate Gibbons edited, formatted and proofed chapters, and created the index. Kate Gibbons coordinated the project. Zeyad Mahmoud and Chiara Pomare wrote the back cover. Jackie Mullins and Sue Christian-Hayes continued to provide excellent administrative support enabling projects under-taken at the Australian Institute of Health Innovation to proceed with ease and the usual high quality.

JB, EH, GH
Sydney, Nivå, Vancouver
September 2020

Editor Biographies

Jeffrey Braithwaite, BA, MIR (Hons), MBA, DipLR, PhD, FIML, FACHSM, FFPHRCP (UK), FAcSS (UK), Hon FRACMA, FAHMS is Founding Director, Australian Institute of Health Innovation; Director, Centre for Healthcare Resilience and Implementation Science; and Professor of Health Systems Research, Faculty of Medicine, Health and Human Sciences, Macquarie University, Australia. His research examines the changing nature of complex health systems, attracting funding of more than AU$145 million (€89 million, £82 million). He has contributed over 640 peer reviewed publications including 14 previous books, and presented at international and national conferences on more than 1,000 occasions, including over 100 keynote addresses. His research appears in journals such as *Journal of the American Medical Association, BMC Medicine, The British Medical Journal, The Lancet, Social Science & Medicine, BMJ Quality & Safety* and *International Journal for Quality in Health Care*. He has received 55 different national and international awards for his teaching and research. Further details are available on the AIHI website: http://aihi. mq.edu.au/people/professor-jeffrey-braithwaite and his Wikipedia entry at https:// en.wikipedia.org/wiki/Jeffrey_Braithwaite.

Erik Hollnagel, MSc, PhD, is Senior Professor of patient safety at Jönköping University (Sweden), Visiting Professorial Fellow at the Centre for Healthcare Resilience and Implementation Science, Macquarie University, Australia, and Professor Emeritus at the Department of Computer Science, University of Linköping, Sweden. Throughout his career he has worked at universities, research centres and industries in several countries and with problems from many domains including nuclear power generation, aerospace and aviation, software engineering, land-based traffic and health care. His professional interests include industrial safety, resilience engineering, patient safety, accident investigation and modelling large-scale socio-technical systems. He has published widely and is the author or editor of 24 books, including five books on resilience engineering, as well as a large number of papers and book chapters. The latest titles are *Safety-I and Safety-II in Practice* and *Working Across Boundaries*.

Garth Hunte, MD, PhD, FCFP is a Clinical Professor and Emergency Physician at Providence Health Care/UBC, a Virtual Physician, HealthLinkBC Emergency iDoctor-in-assistance, the Innovation Lead for Patient Safety and Resilient System Performance in Emergency Care in the Department of Emergency Medicine, University of British Columbia, a scientist at the Centre for Health Evaluation and Outcome Sciences, Providence Health Care Research Institute, a member of the Centre for Health Education Scholarship, and a member of the Physician Advisory Committee, Exceptional Quality, Safety and Value, Providence Health Care, in Vancouver, Canada. His research programmme centres around how safety is created in complex socio-technical systems, and in the application of resilience engineering in healthcare. He is actively involved in the Resilience Engineering Association and the Resilient Health Care Network, and organised/hosted the 6th Resilient Health Care Meeting in Vancouver in 2017.

List of Contributors

Takeru Abe Department of Quality and Safety in Healthcare, Yokohama City University Medical Center, Yokohama, Japan.

Ruth Baxter Bradford Institute for Health Research, Bradford, United Kingdom.

Jeffrey Braithwaite Australian Institute of Health Innovation, Faculty of Medicine, Health and Human Sciences, Macquarie University, Sydney, Australia and International Society for Quality in Health Care (ISQua), Dublin, Ireland.

Elizabeth Buikstra Cairns and Hinterland Hospital and Health Service, Cairns, Australia.

Robyn Clay-Williams Australian Institute of Health Innovation, Faculty of Medicine, Health and Human Sciences, Macquarie University, Sydney, Australia.

Nikki Damen Department of Quality and Safety, Elisabeth-TweeSteden Hospital, Tilburg, The Netherlands and "Tijd voor Verbinding" (National Dutch Safety Programme), Dutch Hospital Association, Utrecht, The Netherlands.

Marit S. de Vos Department of Surgery, Leiden University Medical Center, Leiden, The Netherlands and Department of Obstetrics and Gynaecology, Leiden University Medical Center, Leiden, The Netherlands.

Ellen S. Deutsch Department of Anesthesiology and Critical Care Medicine, The Children's Hospital of Philadelphia, Philadelphia, Pennsylvania and Department of Anesthesiology and Critical Care, University of Pennsylvania Perelman School of Medicine, Philadelphia, Pennsylvania.

Carlos Torres Formoso Post Graduate Program in Construction and Infrastructure, Universidade Federal do Rio Grande do Sul (UFRGS), Porto Alegre, Brazil.

Jaap F. Hamminge Department of Surgery, Leiden University Medical Center, Leiden, The Netherlands.

Erik Hollnagel Hälsohögskolan i Jönköping, Jönköping University, Jönköping, Sweden.

Garth Hunte Department of Emergency Medicine, Faculty of Medicine, University of British Columbia, British Columbia, Canada and Centre for Health Evaluation and Outcome Science (CHEOS), Prvidence Health Care Research Institute, British Columbia, Canada.

Jennifer Jackson Faculty of Nursing, University of Calgary, Calgary, Canada.

Harumi Kitamura Department of Clinical Quality Management, Osaka University Hospital, Osaka, Japan.

Zeyad Mahmoud Australian Institute of Health Innovation, Faculty of Medicine, Health and Human Sciences, Macquarie University, Sydney, Australia and Université de Nantes, Laboratoire d'Economie et de Management de Nantes Atlantique, Nantes, France.

Rie Mieda Department of Anesthesiology, Graduate School of Medicine, Gunma University, Gunma, Japan.

Jenni Murray Bradford Institute for Health Research, Bradford, United Kingdom.

Kazue Nakajima Department of Clinical Quality Management, Osaka University Hospital, Osaka, Japan.

Shin Nakajima Departments of Neurosurgery and General Medicine, National Hospital Organization, Osaka National Hospital, Osaka, Japan.

Kyota Nakamura Department of Quality and Safety in Healthcare, Yokohama City University Medical Center, Yokohama, Japan and Department of Clinical Quality Management, Osaka University Hospital, Osaka, Japan.

Jane K. O'Hara School of Healthcare, Faculty of Medicine and Health, University of Leeds, Leeds, United Kingdom and Bradford Institute for Health Research, Bradford, United Kingdom.

Mary Patterson Center for Experiential Learning and Simulation, Department of Emergency Medicine, University of Florida, Gainesville, Florida.

Natália Ransolin Post Graduate Program in Construction and Infrastructure, Universidade Federal do Rio Grande do Sul (UFRGS), Porto Alegre, Brazil.

Mitchell Sarkies Australian Institute of Health Innovation, Faculty of Medicine, Health and Human Sciences, Macquarie University, Sydney, Australia.

Tarcisio Abreu Saurin Industrial Engineering and Transportation Department, Universidade Federal do Rio Grande do Sul (UFRGS), Porto Alegre, Brazil.

Edward Strivens Cairns and Hinterland Hospital and Health Service, Cairns, Australia and School of Medicine and Dentistry, James Cook University, Townsville, Australia.

Mark Sujan Human Factors Everywhere Ltd, Woking, United Kingdom and Warwick Medical School, University of Warwick, Coventry, United Kingdom.

Makiko Takizawa Department of Healthcare Quality and Safety, Graduate School of Medicine, Gunma University, Gunma, Japan.

Akihiko Yokohama Division of Blood Transfusion Service, Gunma University Hospital, Gunma, Japan.

Part I

Openings

OPENINGS

We begin our sixth volume of Resilient Health Care with two contributions. First, Braithwaite, Hollnagel and Hunte trace the journey through the previous five books in the series, and put the case for turning Lindblom's famous papers on purposeful muddling into an overarching theme for the present volume. In the history of ideas, even at first glance it is clear that resilient health care and muddling with a purpose are close cousins. But what are the more precise similarities – and differences? The editors offer their introductory ideas by way of presaging the chapters that follow.

Second, Hollnagel advances these initial ideas by arguing the point that muddling through is not some kind of option for organisational agents, but an actual necessity. As we will see, this is a point that chapter writers will explicate in many different ways as they present their findings and theories in more detail in the subsequent Parts of the volume (Figure 1).

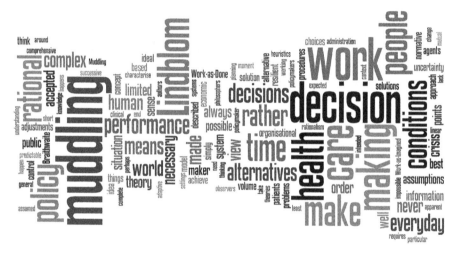

FIGURE 1   A word cloud of Part I. (Source: http://www.wordle.net/)

1 Introduction
How We Got Here

Jeffrey Braithwaite, Erik Hollnagel and Garth Hunte

This is the sixth volume in the Resilient Health Care series. Previous books have provided entry points for extensive discussions on the underlying concepts that we work with in the resilient health care network (https://resilienthealthcare.net/) (e.g., working across boundaries; the resilience of everyday clinical work; Work-as-Imagined and Work-as-Done). On reflection of the intellectual journey we have made to date through the previous volumes, a 'lightbulb' moment happened one day during the early planning stages for this book – namely to use Charles E Lindblom's idea of muddling through as a galvanising paradigm for what people were doing in order to accomplish their work in everyday care settings. We knew that individuals and groups spend much time purposefully navigating through their workplaces, making choices, exercising decisions and solving problems, incrementally – to use another well-worn Lindblomian word – as they face everyday occurrences. And we were convinced it would be worthwhile to explore further.

The research and theory contained in the previous five volumes (Hollnagel, Brathwaite, & Wears 2013, 2019; Wears, Hollnagel, & Braithwaite, 2015; Braithwaite, Wears, & Hollnagel, 2017; Braithwaite, Hollnagel, & Hunte, 2019) have documented the many ways in which people adjust or modify what they do to ensure that work goes well – as it usually does. They do this by dealing effectively with the myriad of minor problems and hassles that work presents, crafting adjustments and adaptations to get things done, and offering solutions to all manner of challenges along the way. Although it may be postulated that people – clinicians, managers, policymakers and patients – simply follow prescribed guidelines and standardised procedures, it is quite apparent that a well-functioning health care system requires all involved to flex and accommodate to circumstances they face minute by minute, hour by hour, day by day.

Although this view has been apparent to seasoned observers of organisational life for many decades, not everyone has made this observation or understood its implications. Many scholars ascribe to more linear, mechanistic views of the world of work. Charles E Lindblom noticed this dichotomy as far back as 1959, and his great insight was that public policymaking necessarily involves a series of successive approximations in contrast to the view of the majority in his scholarly community who held firm to a view that the crafting of policy was best described in a master-planning, strategic, top-down frame. Lindblom saw that imprecision, ambiguity and incrementalism are what is observed when policy is being made, rather than predictable, certain, step-wise, chain logic approaches. Public policymakers are not insightful grand chess masters with the ability to factor in all the variables in pursuit of a perfect endgame. They are normal human beings who try to do the best they can under less-than-perfect circumstances, facing uncertainties, insufficient data, and political, cultural and eco-nomic constraints. Making daily adjustments, taking two steps forward and one back, or tracking sideways on occasion; making trade-offs, and reaching compromises, yet mostly doing well – this is the stuff not only of policymaking, but organisational life at large.

***

To provide context for the present volume, it's worth reflecting on what Lindblom said in his famous first and second papers. In the initial muddling article, Lindblom (1959: *The science of muddling through*) described two methods of policy formula-tion. The first, the root method, is expressed as a 'rational-comprehensive' approach. It is an idealised, normative, staged way of making policy. Using a worked example of a policymaker aiming to control price inflation, he described the rational-mechanical stages as listing values; rating all potential policy outcomes; systematically comparing all alternatives; using theory to describe what should happen; and then after this machine-like, prescribed approach was followed, choosing among alternatives to opti-mise the values he or she started with. The ultimate end points are established at the outset, and the policy is meant to achieve those ends. We now refer to this approach as Work-as-Imagined, or in this case, policy formulation-as-imagined. It can be described *for* but never practised *in* the real world.

To articulate the second method, the 'successive limited comparisons' approach, Lindblom used a branch metaphor. Here, the policymaker sets broad, simple goals to be pursued and ignores many other potential options and variables. Then, the handful of policies that occur to the formulator are outlined and compared. Theory is ignored and instead past empirical examples of policymaking about inflation are considered. The preferred policy option is then chosen, and the process is repeated in order to make incremental gains across time.

While the first is a kind of universal, idealised template for policy design which attempts to be comprehensive and logical, the second is based on trial and error and predicated on mutual adjustments, best guesses and adaptive progress over time. The former specifies the end points and designs the means to achieve the goal: the latter works through the means to achieve acceptable results which are staging points rather than end points.

Lindblom's later paper (1979: *Still muddling, not yet through*) teased out and extended the incrementalist model. Expressed in more detail, the muddling idea is seen as much more akin to the satisficing of Herbert Simon (1947, 1956) by which Simon observed that organisational decision-makers, faced with information defi-cits, complex settings and intractable problems, settle for an option that does the job adequately and reaches a criterion of *acceptability* rather than seek an *optimal* solution which is unrealistic. (Simon assumed this was a consequence of the lim-ited information processing capacity of humans.) In the real-world, optimal solutions do not exist. There are variations on the muddling theme offered in Lindblom's (1979) second paper, and new phrases are introduced, such as non-synoptic incrementalism, limited incremental analysis, and partial mutual adjustment. Each of these fundamentally involves pluralist, multi-stakeholder decision-making in complex organisational ecosystems where trade-offs and compromises are ubiquitous features.

Essentially this branch model describes how policymakers (and by extension other actors in organisations) cope with imprecision and uncertainty, allow themselves space to manoeuvre, make their way in the world in the face of perennial incompleteness, take shortcuts, use best guesses, cope with theirs and others' bounded rationality and exercise degrees of freedom – all in sharp contrast to prescribed, rational planning methods. This phenomenon also resonates with the research of Van de Ven and his analysis of the innovation journey (Van de Ven et al., 1999). That work shows how individuals in and around companies, government agencies and other types of organisations attempt to innovate across time, often entrepreneurially. They shift sometimes from attempting to be rational planners to other times going with the flow and yet other times flying by the seat of their pants, always under conditions of ambiguity, levels of doubt and the vagaries of uncertainty.

***

Having briefly established the ground work and articulated some of Lindblom's core concepts, we now turn to a perspective on how people go about muddling purposefully in health care. Think of people who are trying to make their way in the health care setting in which they work. They might be a health sector policymaker or regulator, formulating procedures and big-picture strategies; a manager with responsibility for a health service, division of a hospital or clinical team; or a clinician at the 'coalface', treating patients in an emergency department, ward or intensive care unit. Indeed they might be anyone who works in the organisation. How can we make sense of what they are doing as they proceed across a shift, as they do their work, striving to contribute to high-quality, safe care for patients who come into the system seeking to have their well-being maintained, their conditions treated, or their symptoms alleviated?

Some would have it (not only before Lindblom but even today) that such health care stakeholders will make rational choices, follow organisationally prescribed ways of doing things, and that the decisions they make can be explained by, for example, formal decision-making theory. Others might say that health care agents will for the most part adhere as well as possible to all the many carefully crafted policy documents, standardised practices or guidelines that are developed, across all health care systems.

A more sociologically grounded account with a debt to Lindblom will see the behaviours of these agents in health care workplaces as more messy, inexact and variable. Those observers will notice people doing complex work in complex settings with limited correspondence to what the policy manual says they should be doing – and limited possibility of actually doing so. People in health care are instead making sense, adapting their behaviour to exigencies, navigating the complex world they inhabit and getting by as best they can, and when they make decisions they do so under conditions of uncertainty and with a lack of good data on which to base their choices.

Under both models, agents will be teleological, goal-orientated and purposeful. But in the first model those describing the in situ agents will be imagining a world that does not actually exist – one that is seen as neatly categorised, robot-like and predictable. In the second condition observers will be seeing the complex, multi-faceted and unpredictable aspects of the world of health care stakeholders. Either world view obviously has consequences for how work is planned, managed, and evaluated.

***

So, following Lindblom's footsteps, we wanted to explicate the notion of muddling with a purpose and use it as a paradigm for the authors of the chapters that follow. We asked our chapter authors in this volume to expand our knowledge of resilient health care, and to do so by paying homage to the concepts Lindblom outlined in those famous papers in 1959 and 1979.

We invited them to examine the contours of the theme 'muddling through with purpose' and to consider its importance in regard to patient safety generally, and resilient health care specifically. We took as our starting position the typical working conditions in health care:

1. health care is an open system;
2. it is a complex adaptive system rather than a linear system;
3. problems and challenges in everyday clinical work are ill-structured;
4. uncertainty is rife, and unresolvable; and
5. resilient performance represents adaptive control in complex systems, i.e., continual adjustment to incrementally satisfy functional goals.

That was the goal of this volume. It is time to turn to reviewing what our authors did when they accepted our invitation to develop their chapter in the light of Lindblom's work.

REFERENCES

Braithwaite, J., Hollnagel, E., & Hunte, G. S. (Eds.). (2019). *Resilient Health Care, Volume 5: Working Across Boundaries*. Boca Raton, FL: CRC Press.

Braithwaite, J., Wears, R. L., & Hollnagel, E. (Eds.). (2017). *Resilient Health Care, Volume 3: Reconciling Work-as-Imagined and Work-as-Done*. Boca Raton, FL: CRC Press.

Hollnagel, E., Braithwaite, J., & Wears, R. (Eds.). (2019). *Resilient Health Care, Volume 4: Delivering Resilient Health Care*. Abingdon, UK: Routledge.

Hollnagel, E., Braithwaite, J., & Wears, R. L. (Eds). (2013). *Resilient Health Care*. Farnham, UK: Ashgate Publishing.

Lindblom, C. E. (1959). The science of 'muddling through'. *Public Administration Review*, 19(2), 79–88.

Lindblom, C. E. (1979). Still muddling, not yet through. *Public Administration Review*, 39(6), 517–526.

Simon, H. A. (1947). *Administrative Behavior: A Study of Decision-Making Processes in Administrative Organization* (1st ed.). New York, NY: Macmillan.

Simon, H. A. (1956). Rational choice and the structure of the environment. *Psychological Review.* 63(2), 129–138.

Van de Ven, A., Polley, D., Garud, R., & Venkataraman, S. (1999). *The Innovation Journey.* New York, NY: Oxford University Press.

Wears, R., Hollnagel, E. & Braithwaite, J. (Eds.). (2015). *Resilient Health Care, Volume 2: The Resilience of Everyday Clinical Work.* Farnham, UK: Ashgate Publishing.

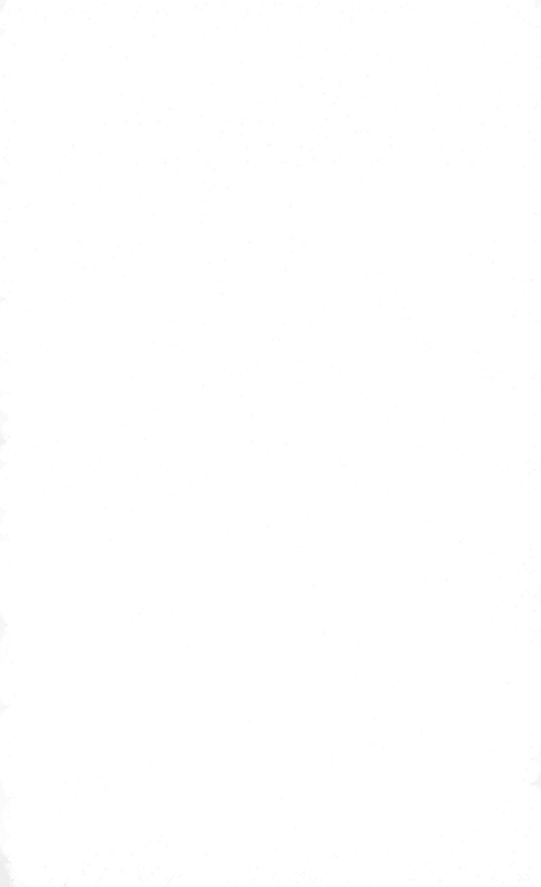

2 The Necessity of Muddling Through

Erik Hollnagel

CONTENTS

INTRODUCTION

In the context of preparing for and managing how socio-technical systems function it is a source of considerable frustration that people – the so-called human factor – often do things differently from what was expected or intended. This occurrence has been given many names, from negatively loaded terms such as deviation and non-compliance to more neutral terms such as adaptations, improvisations, and adjustments. There have also been a number of theories and hypotheses that try to explain why this happens, to say nothing of solutions that promise to get rid of it.

The lack of consistency and uniformity in human performance, the apparent inability to perform as required by the norm, has blithely been accepted as a problem to which a solution should be found. But one might equally well ask whether it is not the norm that is the problem. In other words, why have we – academics and practitioners alike – so willingly accepted the concept that there is an ideal performance, a norm or a standard, that we should strive to achieve? Why do we look at Work-as-Done using Work-as-Imagined as a reference rather than the other way around?

THE HISTORICAL CONTEXT

When Charles Lindblom introduced the concept of muddling through (Lindblom, 1959), the context was administrative decision-making in public administration. The concept was part of the theory of incrementalism in policy and decision-making, the idea that larger, broad-based policy change should be brought about through many small policy changes enacted over time, by successive limited comparisons, rather than by comprehensive strategic thinking and planning. The concept of muddling through is still widely used within the field of public administration but has also been adopted for the study of individual decision-making alongside similar ideas such as *satisficing* (March & Simon, 1958) and naturalistic decision-making (Klein, Orasanu, Calderwood & Zsambok, 1993). Here the problem was that human decision-makers rarely, if ever, were as rational as they should have been according to the theories. Decisions-as-Imagined were represented by normative decision theory, which assumed a decision-maker who was able to analyse and assess a situation with perfect accuracy. Decisions-as-Done were represented by descriptive decision theory, which tried to propose some consistent rules that could account for observed behaviours but still retain the illusion of rationality (Tversky, 1972).

According to the dictionaries, the everyday meaning of 'muddling through' is 'to manage to do something although you are not organised and do not know how to do it'. That was, however, not what Lindblom intended (even though it every now and then is tempting to suspect that it may be true for at least some public administrators). Neither is this negative connotation intended when the term is applied to individual performance and Work-as-Done. Muddling through should not be seen as an indication of incompetence but rather represents the opposite; it is a handy term to characterise the practical solutions that people apply to overcome the inevitable limitations on time, information and possibly other resources that characterise everyday working conditions – in public administration, in health care, and everywhere else.

Logic and Rationalism

It is a consequence of consciousness that we can think about how we think. (Some have even proposed that it is a definition of consciousness and of being human – *cogito ergo sum.*) Philosophers, but by no means philosophers alone, have always been interested both in how we *actually* think and also in how we *should* think. The most famous historical example of that is, of course, the use of Aristotelian logic as the basis for everyday reasoning – for Thinking-as-Imagined. One important legacy of the Aristotelian view is that thinking in general and decision-making in particular is a discrete and identifiable activity or function – rational or 'irrational' as the case may be – carried out by an individual. Later philosophers, notably Descartes, Spinoza and Leibnitz, established the idea of rationalism which assumes that reality has an intrinsically logical structure, that certain truths exist, and that we can grasp these truths by reasoning alone. This developed into the doctrine that human beings are mere automatons or machines (La Mettrie, 1748), a view that centuries later was reinforced and popularised by the onslaught of human information processing (Lindsay & Norman, 1972). (The opposite view of rationalism is empiricism, according to which knowledge primarily is obtained via sensory experiences. Reasoning is therefore not enough.)

Philosophy aside, it is clearly necessary in every situation to be prepared as far as possible for what may happen next. In order to get through the day we continuously need to make sense of the current situation and to anticipate how it could develop. The ability to predict what is going to happen – as well as to make sense of it when it happens – must be based on or refer to a set of assumptions about how the 'world' works, that everyone makes whether they are aware of it or not. Furthermore, most assumptions that work quickly become tacit and blend into the common knowledge, or common sense, we rely on and take for granted. These assumptions apply to what happens around us – why the sun rises, when it will start to rain, why people get ill, how we can safely make a workaround, etc., – and especially include what other people do and are likely to do in specific situations. In the 18th and 19th centuries, when political economists studied how production or consumption were organised in nation-states, it was in particular necessary to understand how people made their decisions and why they would choose one alternative rather than another. In other words, economic philosophers needed a model of how humans make decisions in order to describe how societies functioned. To make a long story short, the result was derived by combining rational thinking and utilitarianism to produce the image of the rational economic decision-maker that is still with us today. The *homo economicus* provided a convenient hypothetical subject, whose narrow and well-defined motives made him – or her – a useful abstraction for the economic and political analyses.

Homo Economicus

It is a fundamental assumption in normative decision-making that people *make* rational decisions and that they *act* rationally because they *are* rational. Being rational means three things in particular. First that the decision-maker knows all alternatives, all possible courses of action, and furthermore knows the outcome of any action taken. Second that the characterisation of alternatives is infinitely divisible. This means that two alternatives never will be identical and also that the decision-maker is able to notice even the smallest differences (a.k.a. infinite sensitivity). Third that the decision-maker can order the alternatives according to a specific preference or criterion so that the alternative which ranks highest can be identified and consequently chosen. In addition to that it is also – tacitly – assumed that the person acts alone and that the conditions or environment are stable – or at least perfectly predictable – during the time it takes to make a decision.

These assumptions about how decisions are made, Decisions-as-Imagined, are unsurprisingly widely acknowledged to be psychologically unrealistic (Peterson & Beach, 1967; Tversky & Kahneman, 1974). It is relative to this ideal that muddling through is useful to characterise Decisions-as-Done. In relation to performance in general, Work-as-Done is accepted because it reluctantly is acknowledged that Work-as-Imagined for several reasons is both misleading and practically impossible. In the same way, except for the reluctance, muddling through should be accepted as a characterisation not only of decision-making but of work in general. Humans simply do not possess the mental faculties that *homo economicus* requires. We can never know or find out about all alternatives, we cannot always distinguish clearly between them, and we are often inconsistent in the criteria we apply and how we use them to make a choice.

THE PRACTICAL CHALLENGES

Altogether this means that muddling through – performance adjustments and performance variability – must be accepted for psychological reasons alone. But even if people were as rational and had the mental or cognitive capacity that the normative theories assume, there are other and perhaps even more compelling reasons why the ideal of decision-making and of human performance is unrealistic. This has to do with the unspoken assumptions about the conditions of work or of the situation on which the ideal is based.

Things take time – and during that time the situation changes. Work-as-Imagined requires a World-as-Imagined where alternatives or possible options do not change while they are being evaluated and perhaps not even after a choice has been made. In the World-as-Imagined there are no windows of opportunity or perhaps rather windows of an infinite size. But in real life opportunities come and go and may exist only for a short time, just as demands may change from moment to moment. That in itself makes it impossible to evaluate alternatives thoroughly.

Information is never just perfect. Information may either be lacking – or time to retrieve it may be in short supply – or it may be in excess, a condition known as information input overload, which means that there may not be time enough to sift through it. People have learned to cope with these conditions by applying a number of powerful heuristics and by trading off thoroughness for efficiency (Hollnagel, 2009). These heuristics, by virtue of being heuristics, usually work but not always. When they fail they are pointed to as evidence of muddling or non-compliance, blissfully ignoring the fact that they represent the rule rather than the exception.

Finally, people are never alone and can never refer only to their personal preferences or criteria. It is always necessary to consider the needs and expectations of others involved – fellow workers, patients, clients, etc. There are many kinds of considerations to be made, to say nothing of the social pressures and expectations from colleagues, management, and society. The bottom line is that muddling through is necessary simply because neither rational decisions nor full compliance are possible.

MUDDLING THROUGH DURING A CRISIS

Despite these facts, the convenience of assuming that performance can be standardised is so strong that most of us rely on it willy-nilly. Muddling through is therefore seen as undesirable for everyday work situations, not least by those who have to prepare and manage them. The irony is that the unreasonableness of this perspective becomes obvious during a crisis. Indeed, a crisis will in itself – and almost by definition – make muddling through necessary simply because the conditions will be so markedly different from the usual that the tried and tested cannot be expected to succeed. In a crisis, strategies are replaced by tactics and tactics may in turn be replaced by opportunistic choices or even trial and error. The usual ways of making decisions and complying with procedures will clearly not work well which leaves muddling through or incremental decision-making as a natural alternative. Yet the conditions during a crisis are basically the same as during everyday work: insufficient time, unexpected events, uncertain future developments competing objectives, and a need to do something before it is too late. The differences are in the magnitude or extent of these conditions, not in their type.

During a crisis, the need to muddle through is further amplified because the surroundings themselves are forced into muddling through, leading to a situation of mutually amplifying deviations or variability (Maruyama, 1963). The solution to that is not to restore order, hence predictability, since a precondition for that is a complete understanding and a complete control that is impossible. Indeed, it is the lack of complete understanding and control that constitutes the preconditions for muddling through. Guidelines and procedures are furthermore never exact because they are themselves affected by the muddling through of planners and designers. (This echoes one of Bainbridge's famous 'Ironies of Automation' (Bainbridge, 1983).) The solution is rather to try to understand the mutual dependencies, since that understanding will provide the predictability that is necessary for more strategic decisions.

The bottom line is that we should not look at muddling through – or Work-as-Done – as an exception that is necessary for people to carry out their work under unusual or unexpected conditions. Instead, we should acknowledge that the conditions always will be different from what has been imagined which means that it is not muddling through, but rather the idolised alternative – rational performance and decision-making – that is an anomaly.

REFERENCES

Bainbridge, L. (1983). Ironies of automation. *Automatica*, 19(6), 775–779.
de La Mettrie, J. O. (1748). *Man a Machine*. Retrieved July 20 2020, from http://bactra.org/LaMettrie/Machine/.
Hollnagel, E. (2009). *The ETTO Principle: Why Things That Go Right Sometimes Go Wrong*. Farnham, UK: Ashgate Publishing.
Klein, G. A., Orasanu, J., Calderwood, R., & Zsambok, C. E. (Eds.). (1993). *Decision Making in Action: Models and Methods*. Norwood, NJ: Ablex.
Lindsay, P. H., & Norman, D. A. (1972). *Human Information Processing*. New York, NY: Academic Press.
March, F. G., & Simon, H. A. (1958). *Organizations*. New York, NY: John Wiley.
Maruyama, M. (1963). The second cybernetics: Deviation-amplifying mutual causal processes. *American Scientist*, 55, 164–179.
Peterson, C. R., & Beach, L. R. (1967). Man as an intuitive statistician. *Psychological Bulletin*, 68(1), 29–46.
Tversky, A. (1972). Elimination by aspects: A theory of choice. *Psychological Review*, 79(4), 281.
Tversky, A., & Kahneman, D. (1974). Judgment under uncertainty: Heuristics and biases. *Science*, 185, 1124–1131.

Part II

Case Studies of Muddling

CASE STUDIES OF MUDDLING

We turn to five chapters, each of which exemplifies the case study approach. Case studies have a rich history in social science, and they have often been used in the Resilient Health Care volumes to understand and bring out the importance of specific resilience issues. In this section of our volume, we open with a case from Mahmoud, Sarkies, Clay-Williams, Saurin and Braithwaite which offers an appraisal of the role of French Scheduling Nurses whose work is key to making their operating theatres run, so far as possible, as intended. It takes us deep into the operating theatre to understand purposeful, incremental social action on the part of the Scheduling Nurses and those with whom they interact, particularly surgeons.

Staying with operating theatres, but moving from France to Japan, Takizawa, Mieda, Yokohama and Nakajima look at hospital procedures for ensuring that blood transfusion goes well after they have been redesigned, moving from a paper-based to a bar-code identification system. The adaptive, and ultimately successful adoption of the new procedures, is a feature of this work.

We remain in hospitals but change focus to emergency medical teams (also known in other countries as medical emergency teams or rapid response systems). Nakamura, Nakajima, Nakajima and Abe look at how such teams in Japan respond to events that occur unexpectedly. This case study examines how the emergency medical team changes its shape, scale and leadership in flexible and adaptive ways. The authors use a metaphor of slime mould to help illuminate the shape-changing nature of the team.

Hamming and de Vos have been studying Mortality and Morbidity meetings in the Netherlands over a period of four years, being especially interested in how the people who attend these meetings learn over time. Typically, in Mortality and Morbidity meetings, the focus is on complications and adverse events – what has gone wrong. But this case study shows how the surgical teams in their meetings began to look at success, too. Hamming and de Vos show how participants in the meetings incrementally improved the way Mortality and Morbidity conferencing occurs. They conclude by

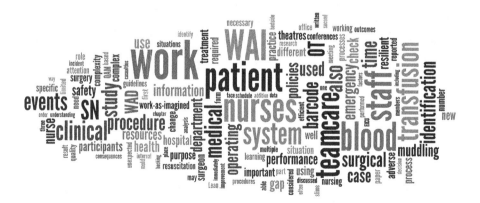

FIGURE 1   A word cloud of Part II. (Source: http://www.wordle.net/)

arguing that the stage they have reached is not the end point, but that further adaptive arrangements will no doubt occur. We are reminded that, as always, improvement is about journeys rather than destinations.

Finally, Jackson draws on her studies in the United Kingdom of nurses and their work, examined through a Resilient Health Care frame. She interviewed 20 nurses, asking them, as they played her video game *Resilience Challenge,* about what they were doing when dealing with the scenarios they encountered while playing the game. Her case study illuminates how nurses explain how they muddle through as they are influenced by Work-as-Imagined expressed in policy documents in order to get things achieved through their everyday clinical work (Figure 1).

3 Managing Complexity and Manifestations of Resilience in Operating Theatres

Sensemaking and Purposive Muddling Among Scheduling Nurses

Zeyad Mahmoud, Mitchell Sarkies,
Robyn Clay-Williams, Tarcisio Abreu Saurin and
Jeffrey Braithwaite

CONTENTS

BACKGROUND

Operating theatres (OTs) are complex environments in which errors or mistakes can quickly escalate and lead to devastating consequences. Despite the widespread proliferation of new organisational models aimed at streamlining processes, standardising actions and increasing predictability (e.g., Lean), achieving performance and safety goals in OTs largely relies on their ability to constantly adapt to varying demands (Mahmoud, 2020). This ability to maintain required operations in the face of unforeseen conditions is commonly referred to as resilience (Braithwaite, Wears, & Hollnagel, 2015).

To be resilient, sociotechnical systems need to continuously monitor their current state, anticipate what may happen in the future, effectively respond to evolving events and integrate learnings from past experiences (Hollnagel, 2011). In health care, the study of resilience has proliferated over the last decade due to recognition of the increasingly complex nature of health organisations (Braithwaite, Clay-Williams, Nugus, & Plumb, 2013; Braithwaite, Wears, & Hollnagel, 2017; Hollnagel, Braithwaite, & Wears, 2013).

In this chapter, we used a qualitative research design to examine resilient performance in action. Drawing on observational data collected in an OT, we focus our attention on the role played by Scheduling Nurses (SNs) in maintaining required performance in the face of an evolving disruption. SNs are tasked with coordinating and ensuring the optimal use of human and material resources to optimise the delivery of safe, efficient and high-quality care. Observing the SNs in action provided a gateway to observe how they muddled with a purpose in achieving their goals (Lindblom, 1959). Our analytical approach was informed by the coping with complexity guidelines proposed by Saurin, Rooke, and Koskela (2013).

The chapter is structured in three sections. In the first section which follows, we introduce our research design and methods. In the next section, we present and analyse the empirical material. Finally, we highlight our findings and discuss them in light of the broader literature on resilience in health care and complexity, paying attention to the notion of purposive muddling (Lindblom, 1959).

RESEARCH DESIGN AND METHODS

Data were collected during a project examining modern managerial practices in OTs (Mahmoud, 2020). Resilient capabilities of the studied organisation were assessed using the guidelines for coping with complexity of Saurin et al. (2013) – see also Bueno, Saurin, Wachs, Kuchenbecker, and Braithwaite (2019).

RESEARCH SETTING

The setting was a public tertiary hospital in France to which we will refer as Grand Lac Hospital (GLH) to preserve its anonymity. GLH is a nationally recognised centre of excellence providing both routine and highly specialised care. This study took place in a newly constructed OT housing 22 operating rooms (ORs) used to conduct elective and emergency surgeries. At the time of the study, the OT was considered a pilot site for deploying new managerial techniques inspired by the Lean management philosophy (Mazzocato, Savage, Brommels, Aronsson, & Thor, 2010). The aim of Lean was to eliminate waste and improve the efficiency of the theatre. It is important nonetheless to note that the OT was functioning in a heavily constrained financial and budgetary environment in which emphasis was placed on the optimum use of productive human and material resources (Mahmoud & Angelé-Halgand, 2018).

RESEARCH DESIGN

The research is reported using a case study framework. Case studies are most appropriate when trying to understand phenomena that are difficult to isolate from their context (Yin, 2014). In accounting for contextual elements, case studies are particularly adapted to our aim of examining how OTs maintain resilience in the face of varying and unforeseen perturbations.

While the data for the broader research project (Mahmoud, 2020) were collected using non-participant observations, semi-structured interviews and document analysis, in this chapter we will draw on observations. In situ real-time observations are particularly useful when studying how organisations react in the face of unforeseen, potentially disruptive events (Journé, 2005).

Although our research design and data collection approach gave primacy to the participants' interactions and the meanings they attributed to them, we were aware of the various subjectivities inherent to this approach characterised by an active participation of the researcher in the data generation and gathering (Wacheux, 1996). To limit bias, we set out to systemise the way we conducted the observations using a three-dimensional matrix (Groleau, 2003). Divided into three columns, not only did the matrix provide space for describing events as they unfolded, but it allowed us to keep track of questions arising during the observations as well as of nascent analytical elements that constituted a first attempt at analysing the data (Table 3.1). The non-constraining nature of the matrix allowed the capturing of a broad range of observed events without limiting our focus, thus enabling a certain opportunism in the face of unfolding events. The opportunistic nature of the observational apparatus is indeed considered key when studying evolving and uncertain situations (Journé, 2005).

A total of 90 hours of observations were conducted, 58 of which took place at the Scheduling Nurses' (SNs') office. The nurses' office was a privileged location for

TABLE 3.1
Three-dimensional data collection matrix (Groleau, 2003)

Date	Observations	Methodological Notes	Analysis Notes
Entry 1	Account of unfolding events as witnessed by the researcher	Annotation of specific events for further inquiry by the researcher (either during another observation session or during another phase of the data collection)	Primary analysis conducted by the researcher during observation sessions (including references to specific research topics or theoretical frameworks)

observing resilient behaviour enacted in the face of emergent complex and unpredictable events.

The SNs played a pivotal role in daily functioning of the OT as they coordinated the pre-, peri- and post-operative logistics required for surgeries to take place. When unanticipated events arose, the nurses had to identify and implement corrective actions to minimise any impact on the OT schedule. In a way, our participants were purposefully muddling through in their tasks as they enacted their role.

DATA ANALYSIS FRAMEWORK

Following their collection, observation field notes were transcribed into narrative episodes each describing a managerial situation, that is a gathering of participants performing a collective action within a defined time and leading to a result subject to external evaluation (Journé & Raulet-Croset, 2008). A theory-informed analysis and coding of the narrative episodes was subsequently conducted using the five guidelines for coping with complexity developed by Bueno et al. (2019). Originating from a review of the literature, these guidelines reflect how organisations manage complexity in their operations as they work towards developing and maintaining their resilience. A succinct summary of the scope of each guideline is provided in Table 3.2.

RESULTS

This section is structured in two parts. First, we present a narrative excerpt of an observational episode conducted at the SN's office. The episode follows a nurse as she tries to mitigate and limit the impact of a potentially disruptive situation. The second part of this section adopts a more analytical lens and discusses the episode in light of the five guidelines for coping with complexity.

TABLE 3.2
Coping with complexity guidelines – adapted from Saurin et al. (2013)

Guideline	Scope
Supporting visibility of processes and outcomes	Systems should promote visibility of complexity, abnormalities and informal work practices.
Organising with slack	To ameliorate tightly coupled processes in order to dampen the consequences of variability.
Encouraging diversity of perspectives when making decisions	Decisions made in complex situations should be informed by complimentary skills of individuals working in teams.
Monitoring and understanding the gap between Work-as-Imagined and Work-as-Done	Gaps between Work-as-Imagined and Work-as-Done should be monitored, questioned, investigated and understood.
Monitoring unintended consequences of improvements and change	Changes of any magnitude interact with each other and with the broader organisational environment. Monitoring those interactions is key to leveraging opportunities and preventing risks.

IN THE EYE OF THE STORM

We are inside the OT, at the SN's office. It is 7:15 am, 45 minutes before the first surgeries are planned to start. Two large screens display the schedule of the 22 ORs. Using a printed copy, the SN highlights patients' names as she receives phone confirmation of their arrival from the reception area located at the opposite end of the 16,000 square metre OT complex. The SN explains that highlighting helps her quickly identify patients that may be late or absent. The start of the operating day is a delicate time, as a disrupted launch of the first cases will not be without consequences on the rest of the day. The SN's role is to orchestrate and optimise the use of resources throughout the day ensuring that the OT schedule is respected.

It is now 10 minutes before surgeries commence. A surgeon (Surgeon A) walks into the office indicating that his name does not appear on the schedule despite him being called in for a first case surgery. The SN checks the schedule, confirms that the surgeon's name is not on it and asks if he could have been mistaken about the date of his surgery. Surgeon A leaves the office, the SN re-examines the printed schedule, and nothing seems to be out of the ordinary. It is now 8:00 am, surgery start time. Surgeon A returns, this time indicating that another surgeon may have originally scheduled the procedure for the patient he is meant to operate on and that he is unable to reach the clinical administration officer who called him last night to inform him of the surgeon change. Surgeon A is only able to provide details on the procedure but cannot recount the patient's name, age or sex and explains that he finds it difficult to remember this information given the large number of patients for whom he provides treatment. Based on the surgery type, the SN was able to identify the patient (Patient X) but explains that the surgery cannot proceed until there is an official confirmation that they have the right patient. The SN calls the booking office to confirm the patient and surgeon's name. Unable to provide an immediate confirmation, the booking staff inform the nurse that they will call again after locating the patient's file.

Shortly after, the SN's phone rings, the OR nursing staff are reporting that the surgeon meant to operate on Patient X is late or absent. The SN explains the situation and says she will call the nursing staff back. Immediately after, the SN calls the OT reception to verify whether the second scheduled patient for that OR has arrived. She explains it might be worth switching these two patients to avoid any further delays as she dials the number of the second patient's surgeon. It is now 15 minutes past the scheduled OR start time. The SN makes the decision to start the second surgery and notifies reception staff and the nurses in the OR to prepare for a new patient. It is after 8:20 am, the booking office returning the SN's call indicates that they could not locate any requests to change the surgeon's name for Patient X. Surgeon A, unhappy with this information, insists that he is meant to operate on Patient X. The SN expresses her confusion as she opens the electronic procedure notes trying to locate any comments or notes that may have been misplaced.

Surgeon A leaves the office. It is now after 8:40 am, Surgeon A returns and passes his phone to the SN. The clinical administration officer on the phone indicates that the surgeon change was due to the withdrawal of the original surgeon. This decision was made after the working hours of the booking office, which is why it was not communicated in time. The surgeon leaves the office furiously howling 'This is unacceptable!'.

MANAGING COMPLEXITY AND MANIFESTATIONS OF RESILIENCE IN THE OT

The narrative episode reveals the importance of the role played by the SN in coping with complexity and maintaining the OT's capacity to perform, despite the emergence of unforeseen and disruptive events (in this case, a last-minute and non-communicated change in the surgical team for one patient). Much like a conductor, the SN orchestrates the execution of a symphony of surgeries harmonising different instruments (staff, patients, equipment) with the aim of staying as loyal as possible to the sheet music (the OT schedule) and keeping the sections of the ensemble (the whole of the theatres) in tune.

The complexity of the task is largely explained by the multiplicity of instruments, or flows, to be harmonised and the fact that some of them are external to the OT, not under the control of the SN (e.g., clinical departments, booking office). As a result, the successful execution of the SN's tasks is dependent on her ability to effectively coordinate a multitude of actors with differing operating methods and priorities. For instance, as described in the episode, the clinical administration officer, representative of a clinical department, successfully resolved the issue of a last-minute withdrawal of Patient X's original surgeon. To avoid cancelling the surgery altogether, the officer identified and reached out to Surgeon A, who agreed to take on the procedure. However, the flow-on effects of this solution were clearly not considered, as the change was not communicated to the OT or the booking office. Beyond a mismatch in priorities, the episode brings to light a broader organisational issue. As revealed during the phone call with the administrative officer, the booking office, the OT and the clinical department have different working hours. This misalignment of work schedules restricts the flow of information between these interdependent entities. The negative consequences of this misalignment were also apparent when Surgeon A wasn't able to reach the administrative officer to confirm the identity of the patient.

The heterogeneity of flows and practices is not only characteristic of processes and entities outside the scope of the OT. In fact, the actors collaborating inside OTs (e.g., surgeons, anaesthetists, anaesthetic nurses, scrub nurses, nurse unit manager and other technical and professional staff), although often described as a team, don't always have the same priorities, strategies or work methods and often have multiple conflicting goals. The SN's capacity to handle the complexity of the work conducted in the OT is the result of a variety of practices and affordances to which we will now turn our attention.

VISIBILITY OF PROCESSES, OUTCOMES AND CONSEQUENCES OF CHANGE

Crucial in supporting the SN's work is an electronic dashboard designed to ensure visibility over the processes taking place in the 22 ORs. The software facilitated real-time performance monitoring and management in a transparent manner. With a glance, the SN was able to see the surgeries scheduled in each of the rooms and monitor their progress in real time. The software was also integrated with numerous other tools that were essential to the nurses' work (e.g., electronic patient records and a centralised patient transport booking system). This software was also used on displays in different areas of the OT, allowing staff to know at a glance the state of the work being conducted.

Beyond its monitoring and tracking capabilities, the software was a fully-fledged decision-support tool presenting the SN with the up to date information (entered by the nurses on the frontline) needed to adapt in real time and thus avoid or minimise the impact of delays and interruptions. This was particularly important given the Lean redesign of the OT, in which processes were tightly coupled, meaning that disruptions often had significant flow-on effects. Such effects were easily visualised digitally when they happened for each of the ORs, using a forecasting capability integrated to the visual management software. This feature also allowed the nurses to monitor the consequences of any planned or unplanned changes to the OT schedule thus maintaining both a micro (action focussed) and macro (system focussed) view of the activities across the OT.

ORGANISING WITH SLACK

In the face of ambiguity or disruptions (e.g., uncommunicated change in the surgical team, missing equipment or surgical complications that require additional OT time), SNs look for ways to minimise, or avoid, unintended consequences that may limit the capacity of the OT to perform adequately. Key to the success of SNs' endeavours was their prerogative to draw upon and properly mobilise a wide range of organisational resources to ensure the continuity of OT operations, despite unexpected events. In our case, the SN was able to contact the clinical department, the booking unit and had access to the patient's medical record. When these resources weren't sufficient, the SN was able to mobilise additional ones, contacting the OT reception, the nursing teams, other surgeons and moving forward another patient's surgery. The availability of these resources broadened our SN's scope of action and thus endowed the OT with the necessary flexibility to adjust when subjected to variability.

DIVERSITY IN DECISION-MAKING

The narrative episode also revealed that the resilient performance of the OT (e.g., anticipate the second surgery, in order to prevent further delays) was largely dependent on the SN's capacity to grasp and structure the various cues surrounding her and subsequently carry out coherent actions. The containment of the incident described above was the result of a multi-stakeholder investigation instigated by the SN as she tried to understand the constitutive dimensions of the unfolding situation. The importance of quickly identifying relevant stakeholders was described as key, especially given the interdependent nature of the tasks carried out by different teams working both inside and outside of the OT. While some of these stakeholders helped articulate the incident (Surgeon A, booking unit, clinical administrative officer) others were partners in the development of an adequate solution (OT reception, nursing staff working in the OR, the surgeon operating on the next patient). Resilient performance in the OT stemmed from the SN's capacity to incorporate a variety of perspectives when trying to sensemake, understand and react to unforeseen events or disruptions.

WORK-AS-DONE AND WORK-AS-IMAGINED

Monitoring the gap between Work-as-Done and Work-as-Imagined was part of our subject SN's role. In addition to the tracking feature implemented in the visual dashboard (discussed earlier), the nurse annotated a printed copy of the OT schedule and highlighted any divergence from the agreed-upon work schedule. The nurse's annotations were usually compiled at the end of the day in a report that complemented the ones automatically generated through the digital dashboard. The nurse's report was described as offering crucial contextual information that not only helped understand why divergences occurred but also how their impact was minimised or mitigated. The SNs together held a weekly meeting with the different nurse unit managers working across the OT to discuss encountered issues and develop strategies to limit their recurrence. Such strategies encompassed changing work practices (Work-as-Done) or modifying work organisations (Work-as-Imagined). These meetings were essential to closing the gap between Work-as-Done and Work-as-Imagined and thus ensuring that staff were well equipped to cope with the complexity of their work.

DISCUSSION

In the OT, resilient performance was the result of multiple practices that included giving visibility to processes and results, organising with slack, considering different perspectives when making complex decisions and monitoring the gap between Work-as-Done and Work-as-Imagined.

This work offers insights into organisational resilience in health care settings. First, the narrative episode presents a unique example of resilient performance in action – or, in the context of this volume of Resilient Health Care, of purposefully and tenaciously muddling through the exigencies of the SN role. It brings to the surface many of the subtleties of the muddling through process (Lindblom, 1959) and thus provides a greater understanding of its inner functioning.

The case study shows how actions and goals are intertwined, and how both must be addressed incrementally when muddling through complex situations. Within the decision-making space, power was distributed between the surgeon and the SN. Their goals were often in conflict and few formal rules existed to govern and coordinate their interactions. In response, the SN practised incremental adjustments; each decision being adapted to the status quo of former decisions. Features of Lindblom's theory of *partisan mutual adjustment* are represented by the fluidity of adjustments, anonymity to system impacts (potential flow-on effects from the SN's response that were not deliberately designed), and recumbent revisiting of decisions based on new information (Lindblom, 1959, 1979; Pal, 2011). The outcomes were achieved as a resultant of partisan mutual adjustment – of 'happening' rather than decided upon. None of the actions taken by the SN were based on premediated rules. Instead, they were improvised on the spot based on the desired goals and evolving situation.

Additionally, from a systems perspective, the study reveals that muddling through at one level, often leads and requires muddling through at another level. First to encounter the incident, the surgeon instigated the process of muddling through, branching out to the SN who subsequently branched out to the booking office and then to other staff working at the OT. Although not visible from the case study, each of these actors arguably engaged in their own process of muddling through as they tried to make decisions and find a solution to the incident.

Moreover, as is typical of muddling through, the case study reveals that although there was a process of bargaining and compromise, it did not necessarily reflect a mutual understanding and alignment of objectives. On one hand, the SN's main priority was to avoid the overflow of the OT and the cost that would be related to that. On the other hand, the surgeon's objective was to find the patient and conduct the surgery, which explains his frustration when that outcome wasn't achieved. The SN and surgeon both derived information and made decisions incrementally. Partisan information was gathered and exchanged, resulting in the prioritisation of different considerations over others. This is another dimension of the muddling through process that was described by Lindblom (1959) in which different parties can agree on the broad course of action to take even though they may diverge on values and goals.

The muddling through lens also reveals insightful knowledge on the use of Lean. The situation described in the case study is likely not to be a rare occurrence in that OT. It is a representation of what happens multiple times throughout the day of the SN. This can't be disassociated from the high level of functional dependencies that characterises Lean organisations. In fact, the role of the SN was specifically created alongside the introduction of Lean in the studied OT. As the case demonstrates, there is a greater need for incrementalism (or muddling through) when processes are tightly coupled, and when interruptions can bring operations to a complete halt. It can be argued that following a rational comprehensive decision-making approach, although feasible, is simply not practical in Lean settings which require agility and timelines when responding to unforeseen events.

In a broader sense, Lean as a philosophy combines both aspects of incremental and rational decision-making. When incidents arise, operators at the sharp end, such as the SN, muddle through to find and implement rapid solutions. It is only in hindsight, when more time is available, that a more comprehensive root-cause analysis of incidents is conducted. At that stage, data are combined from different sources through a systemic and comprehensive process. For example, in the case of the OT, information from the digital dashboard would be combined with the nurse's handwritten annotation and the accounts of other parties involved in the incident. This information would be analysed, and the results of the analysis would inform an action plan aimed at avoiding the reoccurrence of undesirable events. It can therefore be argued that in a Lean and resilient organisation there is a need to combine both incrementalism and rational-comprehensive decision-making. The first of these approaches is a crucial perquisite to adaptability and reactivity in the face of unforeseen events and when rapid action needs to be taken. The second, more comprehensive approach, is more adequate for the purpose of organisational learning and long-term process improvement.

Methodologically, the case study is a testament to the value of using observational and ethnographical research to study resilience. It drew attention to the point that we as researchers were muddling with purpose, not just our subjects. Further, when attending to times of uncertainty, such methodologies can help overcome the limits of traditional retrospective accident analysis approaches that are heavily influenced by multiple biases, most notably that of hindsight (i.e., knowledge of the outcome of a situation at the time of analysis) (Journé, 2013; Woods, 2005).

Our findings have a number of implications for practice: depending on how it is applied, use of Lean methodology, which has been widespread internationally (Mahmoud & Angelé-Halgand, 2018), can enhance or inhibit the ability of OTs to cope with complexity. The Lean principles used in this episode that contributed to coping with complexity were visual management and continuous flow (Liker & Convis, 2005). Over-Leaning a system, however, can make it less resilient, especially where the process removes slack and redundancy from places where they are needed to cope with unexpected events. Lean is not necessarily against slack. It is nevertheless important to ask questions such as: How much slack is needed in dynamic situations? Which types of slack resources? How quickly these can be deployed? What are the system-wide implications of activating slack resources? (Saurin, Rosso, & Colligan, 2017). The replacement of the original surgeon, for example, is a case of slack in this episode. However, this action triggered unintended consequences because the use of the slack resource was not widely communicated to the interested parties. It is possible to design a Lean system with a resilient safety net. However, the more we strip resources from a system, the more critical the role of the humans in the system become – we need to have better teamwork, communication, decision-making skills, mutual support and so on, to be resilient.

A further implication for practice is the importance of recognising functional dependencies (Sundström & Hollnagel, 2011) between departments or other units when designing work. It seems that each unit in our case study developed their Work-as-Imagined without considering interactions with other units. This explains why they had different working hours. There is a need for a broader Work-as-Imagined that stresses interactions between fragmented parts of Work-as-Imagined. The importance of coordination of work processes across boundaries – vertical, horizontal and/or longitudinal – for resilient systems cannot be overstressed (Hegde & Jackson, 2019; Nyssen, 2011).

Finally, when designing systems, it is important that human factor principles be taken into account. We need to think about the role of people in the system, not just the non-human parts. In our case study, the 'tail appeared to be wagging the dog', i.e., the computer system was designed in a way that did not meet the needs of the SN, so the nurse had to print a copy of the OT schedule and highlight/write notes to annotate Work-as-Done. This type of workaround is a typical response to rectifying a gap between Work-as-Imagined and Work-as-Done (Debono et al., 2019). Additionally, while processes were streamlined by taking advantage of technology, the designers did not consider the increased need for teamwork as a consequence. By not considering how all of the staff interact with the technology (not just the SN), the design of the system did not necessarily support resilience and had unintended consequences (e.g., surgeon getting angry at the SN).

CONCLUSION

The aim of this chapter was to examine how OTs maintain resilience in the face of varying and unforeseen perturbations that affect normative patterned behaviours, structures and processes. Analysing our case in terms of the complexity guidelines enabled us to deepen our understanding of the unfolding of resilient performance in situations of ambiguity and uncertainty. By giving visibility to processes and results, mobilising slack, composing with various perspectives and attending to the gap between Work-as-Done and Work-as-Imagined, the SN was able to successfully muddle through with aplomb, despite the challenges, and reduce the impact of the disruption on the overall performance of the OT.

REFERENCES

Braithwaite, J., Clay-Williams, R., Nugus, P., & Plumb, J. (2013). Health care as a complex adaptive system. In E. Hollnagel, J. Braithwaite, & R. L. Wears (Eds.), *Resilient Health Care* (pp. 57–73). Farnham, UK: Ashgate Publishing.

Braithwaite, J., Wears, R. L., & Hollnagel, E. (2015). Resilient health care: Turning patient safety on its head. *International Journal for Quality in Health Care*, 27(5), 418–420.

Braithwaite, J., Wears, R. L., & Hollnagel, E. (Eds.). (2017). *Resilient Health Care, Volume 3: Reconciling Work-as-Imagined and Work-as-Done*. Boca Raton, FL: CRC Press.

Bueno, W. P., Saurin, T. A., Wachs, P., Kuchenbecker, R., & Braithwaite, J. (2019). Coping with complexity in intensive care units: A systematic literature review of improvement interventions. *Safety Science*, 118, 814–825.

Debono, D., Clay-Williams, R., Taylor, N., Greenfield, D., Black, D., & Braithwaite, J. (2019). Using workarounds to examine characteristics of resilience in action. In E. Hollnagel, J. Braithwaite, R. Wears (Eds.), *Resilient Health Care, Volume 4: Delivering Resilient Health Care* (pp. 44–55). Abingdon, Oxon: Routledge.

Groleau, C. (2003). L'observation. Conduire un projet de recherche. Une perspective qualitative. *Editions EMS. Colombelles*, pp. 211–244.

Hegde, S., & Jackson, C. (2019). Resilient front-line management of the operating room floor: The role of boundaries and coordination. In J. Braithwaite, E. Hollnagel, & G. Hunte (Eds.), *Resilient Health Care, Volume 5: Working Across Boundaries* (pp. 103–114). Boca Raton, FL: CRC Press.

Hollnagel, E. (2011). Epilogue: RAG – The resilience analysis grid. In E. Hollnagel, J. Pariès, D. D. Woods, & J. Wreathall (Eds.), *Resilience Engineering in Practice: A Guidebook* (pp. 275–296). Farnham, UK: Ashgate Publishing.

Hollnagel, E., Braithwaite, J., & Wears, R. L. (Eds.). (2013). *Resilient Health Care*, Farnham, UK: Ashgate Publishing.

Journé, B. (2005). Etudier filemanagement de l'imprévu: Méthode dynamique d'observation in situ. *Finance Contrôle Stratégie*, 8(4), 63–91.

Journé, B. (2013). Collecter les données par l'observation. In M.-L. Gavard-Perret, D. Gotteland, C. Haon, & A. Jolibert (Eds.), *Méthodologie de la recherche en sciences de gestion: Réussir son mémoire ou sa thèse* (2nd ed., pp. 165–202). Prais: Pearsons.

Journé, B., & Raulet-Croset, N. (2008). Le concept de situation : contribution à l'analyse de l'activité managériale en contextes d'ambiguïté et d'incertitude. [The Concept of Situation: Contribution to the Analysis of Managerial Activity in Ambiguous and Uncertain Contexts]. *M@n@gement*, 11(1), 27–55.

Liker, J. K., & Convis, G. L. (2005). *The Toyota Way: 14 Management Principles from the World's Greatest Manufacturer*. New York: McGraw-Hill.

Lindblom, C. E. (1959). The science of "muddling through". *Public Administration Review*, 19(2), 79–88.

Lindblom, C. E. (1979). Still muddling, not yet through. *Public Administration Review*, 39(6), 517–526.

Mahmoud, Z. (2020). *Hospital Management in the Anthropocene: An International Examination of Lean-based Management Control Systems and Alienation of Nurses in Operating Theatres*. (Doctor of Philosophy Thesis, Université de Nantes, France and Macquarie University, Australia) (in press).

Mahmoud, Z., & Angelé-Halgand, N. (2018). L'industrialisation des blocs opératoires : Lean Management et réification. *Management & Avenir Santé*, 3(1), 73–88.

Mazzocato, P., Savage, C., Brommels, M., Aronsson, H., & Thor, J. (2010). Lean thinking in healthcare: A realist review of the literature. *BMJ Quality and Safety*, 19(5), 376–382.

Nyssen, A. S. (2011). From myopic coordination to resilience in socio-technical systems. A case study in a hospital. In E. Hollnagel, J. Paries, D. Woods, & J. Wreathall (Eds.), *Resilience Engineering in Practice: A Guidebook* (pp. 219–235). Farnham, UK: Ashgate Publishing.

Pal, L. A. (2011). Assessing incrementalism: Formative assumptions, contemporary realities. *Policy and Society*, 30(1), 29–39.

Saurin, T. A., Rooke, J., & Koskela, L. (2013). A complex systems theory perspective of lean production. *International Journal of Production Research*, 51(19), 5824–5838.

Saurin, T. A., Rosso, C. B., & Colligan, L. (2017). Towards a resilient and lean health care. In *Resilient Health Care, Volume 3: Reconciling Work-as-Imagined and Work-as-Done*. (pp. 3–17) Boca Raton, FL: CRC Press.

Sundström, G., & Hollnagel, E. (2011). The importance of functional interdependencies in financial services systems. In E. Hollnagel, J. Paries, D. Woods, & J. Wreathall (Eds.), *Resilience Engineering in Practice: A Guidebook*. Surrey, UK: Ashgate Publishing.

Wacheux, F. (1996). *Méthodes Qualitatives et Recherche en Gestion*. Paris: Economica.

Woods, D. D. (2005). Creating foresight: Lessons for enhancing resilience from Columbia. In W. H. Starbuck & M. Farjoun (Eds.), *Organization at the Limit: Lessons from the Columbia Disaster*: Oxford: Blackwell Publishing.

Yin, R. (2014). *Case Study Research: Design and Methods* (5 th ed.). Los Angeles, CA: SAGE.

4 Re-designing the Blood Transfusion Procedure in Operating Theatres
Aligning Work-as-Imagined and Work-as-Done

Makiko Takizawa, Rie Mieda, Akihiko Yokohama and Kazue Nakajima

CONTENTS

INTRODUCTION

The mainstream approach to patient safety, which focusses on the things that go wrong and aims to reduce the number of errors to zero, needs to be changed (Braithwaite, Wears, & Hollnagel, 2015; Hollnagel, 2014). Standardised health care processes as well as the many policies and regulations that have been put in place to reduce errors – which are, in fact, comparatively rare – have been designed according to safety models developed between 1960 and 1980. Rather than focussing on adverse events, contemporary approaches to safety focus on success, and attempt to understand the practice of health care in a wider context.

Blood transfusion is generally considered to be a safe and reliable procedure (Amalberti, Auroy, Berwick, & Barach, 2005) with the rate of incorrect blood type transfusion error as low as 10^{-5} to 10^{-6}. Though the numbers show the procedure's high reliability, blood transfusion in everyday clinical work is not always a static or stable process. According to international research, 70%–80% of adverse incidents occur in clinical areas during pre-transfusion under time pressure and are most frequently the result of identification errors (Fujii et al., 2009; Stainsby, Russell, Cohen, & Lilleyman, 2005). Blood transfusion scenarios can vary greatly – from planned transfusions given in calm environments to those required during emergency procedures. Health care providers are expected to judge situations correctly, often under time pressure and with limited information, in profoundly fluid and uncertain conditions. There is always a trade-off between thoroughness and time efficiency in such emergent settings. Figure 4.1 shows the dynamics of blood transfusion in operating theatres, including the trade-off between procedural thoroughness and time efficiency.

Gunma University Hospital, located in Tokyo's metropolitan area, is an academic hospital with 731 beds. It serves local patients from Gunma and nearby prefectures, and performs approximately 2,200 inpatient surgical operations per year.

In the hospital, we experienced an incident case suggesting a violation of the hospital-wide safety protocol for blood transfusion identification. Instead of only trying to identify a reason for the particular case and blindly enforcing the protocol, we decided to go to the *genba* ('actual workplace'). We observed how blood components are actually being transfused in operating theatres in order to understand the

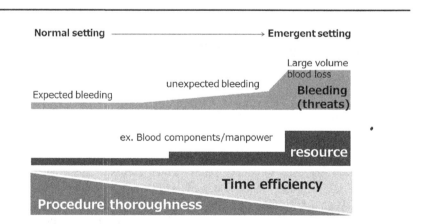

FIGURE 4.1   Dynamics of blood transfusion in operating theatres

practical reality of everyday work – or 'Work-as-Done' – and to identify whether there was any gap between Work-as-Imagined and Work-as-Done.

In this chapter, we describe how muddling through decisions were made by the people behind Work-as-Done. Furthermore, we will discuss how to reconcile the gap between Work-as-Imagined and Work-as-Done.

AN INCIDENT REPORT AND WORK-AS-IMAGINED – WORK-AS-DONE

AN INCIDENT REPORT

The Department of Healthcare Quality and Safety of Gunma University Hospital received an incident report suggesting that a barcode identification was not used immediately before a specific blood transfusion. An unused blood component marked as 'used' in the hospital information system was returned to Blood Transfusion Division Misidentification. Hospital policy for blood transfusion procedures – or 'Work-as-Imagined' – demand the use of barcode identification immediately before transfusion.

WORK-AS-IMAGINED (HOSPITAL-WIDE RULES)

The Gunma University Hospital blood transfusion policy requires ordering, dispensing and safety checking through the hospital information system (HIS) using barcode identification for the blood component lot number and patient wrist band identification (ID) tag. When a patient needs a blood transfusion, a doctor orders blood component products through the HIS. The technician from the Division of Blood Transfusion Service will perform a blood test and prepare for the transfusion. Then, three safety checks are made prior to blood transfusion. The first is made when the blood component products are being dispensed, the second while preparing for the blood transfusion procedure, and a third is made at the patient's bedside immediately before the transfusion. During each verification, staff are required to double check the patient's name, ID number, blood type, lot number, expiration date, irradiation status and the result of cross-matched blood testing. In addition to the physical confirmation, barcodes are also used to match the particulars of each transfusion, blood test and lot number with the patient. The first and second checks are made to confirm the order for the patient, blood test and the lot. The last bedside check, which is the only opportunity that includes patient identification, is the final chance to avoid a potentially fatal mis-transfusion.

In wards and outpatient departments of Gunma University Hospital, physicians order the blood through the HIS, but all other processes that involve dispensing, preparing and transfusing are handled by nurses.

WORK-AS-DONE (OPERATING THEATRES EVERYDAY PRACTICE)

Staff of the Department of Healthcare Quality and Safety visited operating theatres, observed how the work was performed, and interviewed health care providers – mainly anaesthesiologists and the nurses responsible for the actual blood transfusion.

Surgeons order the required blood component products several days before an operation through HIS, and anaesthesiologists decide the timing of the transfusion during the operation. When we visited the *genba* operating theatres, we found that one anaesthesiologist was using a paper form to request blood components dispensing during the surgery. This procedure was unique in the operating theatres and the paper forms were used to share information between the nurse and anaesthesiologist about which blood units were requested for dispensing. According to the request sheet, the nurse called the blood transfusion service for dispensing. The first safety check was performed between the Blood Transfusion Service technical staff and the operating theatre nurse, the second safety check was performed between the operating theatre nurse and the anaesthesiologist both using the paper form and HIS. But for the bedside check immediately before transfusion, which requires patient identification, we noticed that the wrist band ID tag of the patient was covered under the sterile drape at the bedside, which meant that the barcode was difficult to access and use for identification. In the theatre, the anaesthesiologist physically confirmed the blood components and patient name with the paper form for the third check. Barcode-identification for the third check was sometimes performed after the operation by the theatre nurse.

But after observing several operating theatres, we found that in some cases patient wrist bands were cut to introduce an arterial line for continuous blood pressure monitoring; indeed, wrist bands were cut in most of the major surgeries that required blood transfusion.

MUDDLING THROUGH DECISION AND ITS REASONS

BLOOD TRANSFUSION POLICY

Blood transfusion is highly regulated by the government. Both blood component products and blood transfusion processes are detailed in the 'Guideline for blood transfusion therapy' by the Ministry of Health, Labour and Welfare (Ministry of Health, Labour and Welfare, 2005). Each hospital is required to develop their own policies and procedures for blood transfusion in accordance with the guidelines, and health care providers must follow them. To prevent the wrong blood type transfusion, which is considered a 'never event', all the hospital staff are asked to strictly follow the rules.

Identification systems that use barcode technology to avoid errors (Poon et al., 2010) have been implemented in many large Japanese hospitals since 2008. These systems identify patients through barcoded wristband ID tags that are matched to subscribed transfusion medicines and/or blood components. While the high expectations that accompanied the technology have largely been met, like all human systems they are susceptible to misuse and error, and some problems remain (Ahrens, Pruss, Kiesewetter, & Salama, 2005; Ohsaka, Kobayashi, & Abe, 2008; Japan Council for Quality Health Care, 2016). That the sharp-end use of new technology does not always work as imagined, but is disrupted by varying situations, suggests a discrepancy between Work-as-Imagined and Work-as-Done. These gaps can be a result of unwanted over adjustment of the frontline staff and could result in unstable and excessive fluctuations to the process leading to an unexpected hazardous outcome.

The barcode identification system was introduced to Gunma University Hospital as an administrative decision and hospital policies and procedures were developed by management based on ward procedures rather than considering the patterns of practice in operating theatres. The whole blood transfusion procedure including ordering, dispensing and bedside check was thought to be able to be completed without paper forms and thus be safer and more efficient. This was true for most of the hospital but in operating theatres, the staff had difficulty using the barcode system for bedside identification and the system did not work as intended. We recognised this gap between Work-as-Imagined and Work-as-Done through the *genba* visit.

Theatre staff had to 'muddle through' and modify the system to make it work in the theatre context, using paper forms for years. They used both paper forms for physical identification and barcode identification through HIS to fulfil the needs of all the staff, which was safety, keeping track of blood component use and payment. As a result, the procedure in the operating theatre became complex and less efficient.

UNINTENDED FEEDBACK

The barcode system is also used for identifying the actual use and the payment system calculates the costs of blood components and other transfusion medicines. The third check before blood transfusion was not only used for safety purposes but also to identify the actual use. This dual-purpose function of the barcode identification system led to misunderstanding and confusion of some nursing staff. When nurses transfuse the ordered blood but fail to use the barcode system, the billing department is unable to determine whether the ordered blood was unused or has perhaps been misidentified. Then the billing department will call the nurse to ask if they have used it or not. This led some nursing staff to assume that the barcode system was needed for billing purposes but not for patient safety identification especially because they were also using paper forms and physical identification for safety checks.

RECONCILING THE GAP

ROUND TABLE DISCUSSION

A multidisciplinary working group consisting of anaesthesiologists, theatre nurses, quality and safety staff and blood transfusion department staff was convened to discuss the blood transfusion procedures in operating theatres.

PERCEPTION OF THE PRESENT PROCEDURE

Before the barcode identification was introduced, the blood transfusion safety check was performed using paper slips in the hospital. When the barcode identification was introduced, operating theatre staff noticed the difficulties of using the patient wrist band which was covered under the drape and they tried to continue with the paper method. Each professional had different perceptions and opinions about the procedure. Some typical opinions of each professional are shown in Table 4.1.

TABLE 4.1
Typical opinions of different professionals

Anaesthesiologist
  Time efficiency is important as we need to be prepared for an emergency
  We care about safe blood transfusion and double check intensively with the nurse when preparing
  Filling in the paper form takes too much time
  Unfamiliar with barcode identification system and sceptical about its use
Nurses
  The paper form is needed to keep track of the blood component use
  We double check with the anaesthesiologist when preparing
  The billing department will call us if we don't use the barcode system so we do it after the operation
Blood technicians
  Barcode identification immediately before transfusion is essential for safety and also it is faster if
    you get used to it
  Using both paper and the hospital information system is redundant and unnecessary
  Person-machine double check can replace person-person double check
  The system allows to keep track of the blood component use if used for the bedside check

Time efficiency is always a concern for anaesthesiologists, as they are frequently required to make urgent decisions during surgery. Operational procedures are under the control of the surgeon, but the anaesthesiologist is in charge of maintaining the patient's vital signs in response to the evolving surgical process. Additionally, transfusions are often required when the surgery is in its most intense phase, and anaesthesiologists must conduct multiple tasks (including administrating the vasopressor and transfusing liquid) simultaneously to maintain the stability of patients' vital signs. Anaesthesiologists, who were not aware that the written form existed only in the operating theatres, felt that filling in the request form was not a time efficient process.

The operating theatre nurses preferred the paper request form, as they needed to grasp the exact use of the blood components and were afraid of losing track of them. The form was used only for administrative purposes while the actual order was made through the HIS by the surgeons. The dispensing process was electronically processed by the technical staff of the blood transfusion department. The bedside safety check was also able to be processed if the barcode identification system was used as it acted as a safety check enabling the identification of used and un-used blood units. This meant efficient use of the system at the bedside check by anaesthesiologists was adversely affecting the work of nurses which was to keep track of the used and unused blood for records and payment calculation. Furthermore, the barcode was regarded by some nurses as a payment device rather than a safety measure due to the feedback from the billing department.

Technical staff from the blood transfusion department emphasised the importance of barcode use immediately before the transfusion, pointing out that this final check provides the only opportunity to confirm patient identification. They highlighted the benefits of barcode identification in terms of time efficiency and effectiveness, and explained that all staff members use them in other areas of the hospital. They also informed the group that the inspection and accreditation guidelines of the Society of

Transfusion Medicine and Cell Therapy in Japan allows the machine–person double check instead of person–person double check.

CREATING CONSENSUS THROUGH SHARED VALUE

Every staff member was conscientious about the importance of blood transfusion safety and willing to participate in discussion about the procedure and to change it if necessary.

The working group discussion clarified the meaning of each procedure and how their task was connected to each other's task. Through this discussion process, they became aware of redundancy of the request sheet, and highlighted the fact that many theatre staff – both nurses and anaesthesiologists – didn't thoroughly understand the significance of the check immediately before transfusion, which was the only chance to match with the patient, regarding it as more important than the second check preparing for transfusion. The working group agreed that they valued safe and efficient procedure and the appropriate extensive use of the barcode system could help them all fulfil their goals.

As a result of the working group discussion, all participants better understood the blood transfusion procedure and agreed to reorganise the procedure with shared value which was to maximise time efficiency and patient safety. To implement these reforms, it was agreed that the barcode would be used immediately before transfusion, and the paper request form would be eliminated.

The new procedure is as follows:

1. The anaesthesiologist is to call the blood transfusion department directly instead of asking the nurse to make the request using the paper form. The paper form was abandoned.
2. Wristband ID tags are to be cut before the operation and to be used for patient identification at the bedside by the anaesthesiologist. (It will be cut anyway when introducing the arterial line).
3. Machine (barcode)–person check is to be utilised for the bedside check, replacing person–person double check by the nurse and anaesthesiologist.
4. Wristbands are to be refitted post-operatively using the World Health Organisation surgical safety check list (Haynes et al., 2009).

QUESTIONNAIRE SURVEYS

Staff perceptions of the effectiveness of the intervention were gauged through a structured self-evaluation questionnaire survey of anaesthesiologists and theatre nurses 3 and 12 months after the introduction of the new procedure.

We asked anaesthesiologists how frequently they used the barcode identification system immediately before blood transfusion. Their self-evaluated performance had significantly improved: rising from 18% before the intervention, to 53% and 68%, respectively, 3 and 12 months after the intervention (Figure 4.2). Moreover, a majority (73%) of anaesthesiologists evaluated the new procedure as being more efficient and involving less work for them. Forty-four percent of nurses evaluated the new

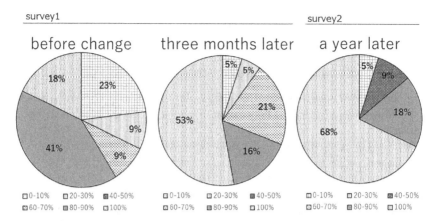

FIGURE 4.2 Questionnaire survey showed improved use of the barcode system by anaesthesiologists

procedure as more efficient, while 39% regarded it as cumbersome. Some nurses reported that anaesthesiologists did not always tell nurses which blood components they had to dispense, a lapse that needed to be improved. In addition, some nurses were concerned about cutting the wristband. These results were revealed to the operating theatre staff after the survey.

EDUCATIONAL VISIT

The Department of Healthcare Quality and Safety also held an educational visit to the anaesthesiology department 3 months after the new procedure was implemented and gave a short lecture to the staff to explain the objectives and rationale behind the change. Additionally, the risk manager of the anaesthetic department played an important role in educating junior doctors when they arrived and began their practice.

DISCUSSION

In this chapter, we described

- How the administrative decision of introducing a barcode identification system affected the practice in operating theatres under restrictions of an access to patient ID.
- How people in the frontline made 'muddle through' decisions, or adaptations, to pursue their tasks depending on their own discretion and priorities which was different among multiple professionals.
- As a result of adjustments, how blood transfusion procedures in the operating theatres became unique and complicated with a mixture of old and new methods.
- How we aligned the gap between Work-as-Imagined and Work-as-Done and showed quantitative data demonstrating how it was accepted by the staff over time.

We showed how the introduction of new technology affected the work of frontline staff in unintended ways, how they managed to pursue their own tasks and created a tangled procedure due to the technical difficulties encountered in the real world, and how it went unresolved for years. Round table discussion revealed how we don't understand each other's tasks and priorities but how we share the value of safe and efficient procedures, and how our tasks are connected to each other. This understanding helped align the gap between Work-as-Imagined and Work-as-Done and re-designed the blood transfusion procedure in the operating theatre under shared values. The new procedure was accepted by health care providers and the rate of barcode identification of patient ID significantly improved over a year.

Barcode use is designed to reduce the effects of human error, and is also used as a low-cost solution to tracking and identifying blood products; however, the optical nature of the system means that there are challenges when visibility is obstructed. Weaknesses in the barcode identification system that were evident when drapes were used to cover the patient's ID meant that certain adjustments were required.

Optical identification systems have limitations not only in operating theatres but can be problematic in other contexts – in dimly lit wards at night, for instance, or when a sleeping patient tucks their arm beneath the bedding. Though barcode identification is still widely used in most departments of the hospital, non-optical systems such as radiofrequency identification (RFID) or other new technology needs to be considered in the health care system.

Also, the dual-purpose barcode system can cause confusion, particularly because of the feedback loop generated by billing issues. Many nurses assumed that the barcode was exclusively billing-related rather than additionally providing a patient identification safeguard, and this misunderstanding was reinforced by calls from the billing department.

Increased understanding of the purpose of the procedure and the role each professional led to the awareness of the values they share and a successful re-design of the blood transfusion procedure in operating theatres.

Our study is an example of muddling through with decisions being made at multiple levels. The administrative level decided to introduce barcode identification to the hospital, management level decided to make a policy related to blood transfusion for the entire hospital, frontline staff level in the operation theatre had to circumvent the physical difficulties of this system. All the decisions made were connected and affected each other and resulted in unintended consequences which was the gap between Work-as-Done and Work-as-Imagined. We also discussed that if the gap is to be reconciled, it is essential that all relevant professionals come together and re-design the new procedure under mutual understanding and a shared value.

This study illustrates the need for careful observation at the *genba*, the actual place, especially when introducing a new system. While individual staff generally adapt to the situation if there are obstacles, explanations and discussions regarding the objectives and the rationale of the system helps align Work-as-Done and Work-as-Imagined, this may, in turn, lead to more efficient and safer procedures under shared values.

REFERENCES

Ahrens, N., Pruss, A., Kiesewetter, H., & Salama, A. (2005). Failure of bedside ABO testing is still the most common cause of incorrect blood transfusion in the Barcode era. *Transfusion and Apheresis Science*, 33(1), 25–29.

Amalberti, R., Auroy, Y., Berwick, D., & Barach, P. (2005). Five system barriers to achieving ultrasafe health care. *Annals of Internal Medicine*, 142(9), 756–776.

Braithwaite, J., Wears, R. L., & Hollnagel, E. (2015). Resilient health care: Turning patient safety on its head. *International Journal for Quality in Health Care*, 27(5), 418–420.

Fujii, Y., Shibata, Y., Miyata, S., Inaba, S., Asai, T., Hoshi, Y., ... Sagawa, K. (2009). Consecutive national surveys of ABO-incompatible blood transfusion in Japan. *Vox Sanguinis*, 97(3), 240–246.

Haynes, A. B., Weiser, T. G., Berry, W.R., Lipsitz, S. R., Breizat, A. H. S., Dellinger, E. ... Gawande, A. A. (2009). A surgical safety checklist to reduce morbidity and mortality in a global population. *New England Journal of Medicine*, 360(5), 491–499.

Hollnagel, E. (2014). *Safety-I and Safety-II. The Past and Future of Safety Mangement.* Farnham, UK: Ashgate Publishing.

Japan Council for Quality Health Care. (2016). *Blood Transfusion to Wrong Patient (1st Follow-up Report).* Tokyo, Japan: Japan Council for Quality Health Care. Retrieved September 7 2020, from http://www.med-safe.jp/pdf/No.110_MedicalSafetyInformation.pdf.

Ministry of Health, Labour and Welfare. (2005). *Guideline for Blood Transfusion Therapy.* Tokyo, Japan: Ministry of Health, Labour and Welfare. Retrieved September 7 2020, from https://www.mhlw.go.jp/new-info/kobetu/iyaku/kenketsugo/5tekisei3a.html.

Ohsaka, A., Kobayashi, M., & Abe, K. (2008). Causes of failure of a barcode-based pretransfusion check at the bedside: Experience in a university hospital. *Transfusion Medicine*, 18(4), 216–222.

Poon, E. G., Keohane, C. A., Yoon, C. S., Ditmore, M., Bane, A., Levtzion-Korach, O., ... Gandhi, T. K. (2010). Effect of bar-code technology on the safety of medication administration. *New England Journal of Medicine*, 362, 1698–1707.

Stainsby, D., Russell, J., Cohen, H., & Lilleyman, J. (2005). Reducing adverse events in blood transfusion. *British Journal of Haematology*, 131, 8–12.

5 Dynamic Performance of Emergency Medical Teams as Seen in Responses to Unexpected Clinical Events

Kyota Nakamura, Kazue Nakajima,
Shin Nakajima and Takeru Abe

CONTENTS

INTRODUCTION

Daily clinical work in the emergency department requires a balance between the available resources and the work necessary to save patients' lives. Supply of key resources (e.g., beds, equipment and doctors) is often limited and changes over time. Factors that determine workload, such as patients' conditions, also change dynamically. Especially when dealing with unexpected events, emergency medical teams must exhibit resilience by responding flexibly and adaptively to these unstable situations. In some ways, this has parallels with what Lindblom called 'muddling through' (Lindblom, 1959, 1979).

To elucidate the team dynamics that promote resilience, we examined the performance of emergency medical teams responding to a mass casualty incident.

CONTEXT

As a tertiary medical institution, our hospital provides emergency response for the most severely ill patients. The emergency department has three resuscitation beds, enabling the clinicians to deal simultaneously with three severely ill patients. On the night shift, which starts at 5:30 pm, three doctors and several junior residents are present. Doctors in internal medicine, surgery, anaesthesia, general intensive care unit (GICU), stroke centre and cardiovascular centre also work on the night shift. Our critical care centre operates an emergency intensive care unit (EICU) with 12 beds and a step-down unit (SDU) with 8 beds.

CASE STUDY: RESPONSE TO MULTIPLE CASUALTIES

Typically, emergency medical teams often experience situations in which they must respond to a few critically ill patients at the same time. On the other hand, when they are forced to respond to a large number of critical patients simultaneously due to a local disaster, it is important to adopt a flexible response by appropriately utilising limited resources (staff, location and equipment).

CONTACT FROM THE AMBULANCE DISPATCH CENTRE

At 6:30 pm on a weekday, a patient with suspected stroke had undergone initial medical treatment on a resuscitation bed in the emergency department. At 6:50 pm, the Ambulance Dispatch Centre reported that multiple casualties, including several casualties with an altered level of consciousness, were incoming following a traffic accident on the highway.

PREPARATION FOR RECEIVING CASUALTIES (STAFF, PLACE AND EQUIPMENT)

Although information was limited, preparation of the emergency department was initiated. First, we arranged for an additional resuscitation bed to be located next to the resuscitation space that is normally used for storage, which meant we had a total of four resuscitation beds for severely injured patients. At the time, the EICU had two empty beds, and it was expected that there would be a shortage of beds available to accept the injured casualties. We asked the GICU, which normally manages in-hospital critically ill and post-operative patients, to receive the stroke patient and to act as backup if it became difficult to secure a vacant bed in the EICU. To secure the available beds in the EICU, we asked the EICU nurse to list candidates for transfer from EICU to SDU. We also informed the surgery department about the possibility of urgent operations.

Next, to secure staff, we asked the emergency, nursing and radiation departments to put staff, who had not returned home, on standby. In addition, based on the information that there were multiple casualties with an altered level of consciousness due to trauma, we requested support from neurosurgery, orthopaedics and anaesthesiology. In preparation for the upcoming patient surge, we planned to place a generous number of medical staff in the resuscitation room. Regarding the allocation of nurses in the resuscitation room, where a shortage of manpower was expected, we asked for support from the nursing department; in addition, the surgical nurses, who were experienced in normal clinical situations, came to support us.

UNEXPECTED PATIENT

At 7:10 pm, a hotline call from an ambulance asked us to receive a 70-year-old male suffering from shock. All staff members believed that the hotline call had come from the accident scene, but in fact it was a different call regarding a different patient who had suspected sepsis.

We immediately decided that it would be necessary to adjust our treatment approach. The initial treatment strategy for this patient with septic shock was to perform only minimal evaluation and first aid in the resuscitation room, and then to admit the patient to the EICU to subsequently perform all other tests and treatments normally, rather than to the resuscitation room. In other words, we decided to use an EICU bed as the fifth resuscitation bed for initial treatment. At the same time, staff assignments were reconsidered, and the surgical team decided to leave the allocation of staff as is in the resuscitation room, while assembling another treatment team without surgeons for treatment of sepsis patients in the EICU. In addition, we asked the EICU nurse to proceed with a plan to secure the available admission beds in the EICU, based on the list of candidates for leaving the ICU.

RECEIVING THE CASUALTIES

In normal clinical practice, patients are treated by a team, which is an aggregation of multiple doctors' experiences and specialties. However, because many doctors who do not usually treat patients together came to provide support, we assembled four temporary treatment teams. Each team consisted of four doctors, considering their limited collaborative experience; one doctor was assigned to be the sub-leader, and was appointed to lead the treatment of the patient.

Initially, we set an overall priority on saving the patient's life, and the initial treatment of each case was determined according to the initial trauma treatment protocol under the sub-leader. When it was necessary to set priorities among multiple cases, such as the order of computed tomography (CT) examinations, a decision was made by the leader based on monitoring of the overall situation in the resuscitation room.

At 7:40 pm, the first casualty who was triaged as red (priority 1: requiring immediate treatment) arrived, and initial treatment was started. Five minutes later, the second casualty triaged as yellow (priority 2: requiring urgent treatment) was delivered, followed by the third casualty, who had been triaged as yellow. Finally, 12 minutes later, the triaged-black (deceased) casualty arrived with the on-site medical team. Considering the overall arrangement of the patients in the resuscitation room, the triaged-black casualty was treated in the temporary resuscitation bed, while the other three casualties were treated in the normal resuscitation beds.

FROM INITIAL TREATMENT TO DEFINITIVE CARE

As assessments and treatments progressed, the details of the casualties became gradually clearer, the number of staff assigned to a casualty with minor injuries decreased, and the staff gathered for the seriously injured casualties. In addition, the allocation was changed so that a neurosurgeon was in charge of a case suspected of head trauma, and an orthopaedic surgeon was in charge of a case with a suspected limb fracture. At this point, we moved into the early phase of definitive care, in which specialised interventions could be performed. As the situation normalised, some of the staff who had initially gathered to help became free and left the resuscitation room and returned to their departments or went home. This included some staff who had been asked to assume roles other than on-site medical care, such as acting as medical photographer. Eventually, except for one patient who was transported in a state of cardiopulmonary arrest, the remaining stroke and sepsis patients, as well as the three other trauma cases, were treated and admitted to the EICU.

FLEXIBLE TEAM RESPONSE TO THE UNEXPECTED CLINICAL EVENT

As we described above, the emergency medical team, when it deals with an unexpected number of casualties, dynamically performs multi-objective optimisation through a complex trade-off of patient factors, medical resources and treatment levels (Figure 5.1). From the preparation to initial treatment phase, large numbers of medical resources are prepared through rough estimations of patient factors based on limited information, whereas our treatment goal was just saving the lives of the patients. Patient factors (number, severity and injury) become clearer as medical treatment progresses, medical resources gradually become more suitable for each patient through repeated fine adjustments, and the treatment level is shifted such that definitive care is provided by a physician with the appropriate specialty. This flexible and autonomous change in organising the team is analogous to the way slime moulds efficiently solve complex problems.

The movements of the emergency medical team can be regarded as a complex set of trade-offs involving medical resources, number and severity of patients, and levels

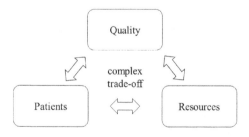

FIGURE 5.1 Multi-objective optimisation by the emergency medical team

of medical treatment. Initially, the goal of medical treatment is to save lives based on the balance between medical resources and patient factors. Subsequently, while repeatedly performing fine adjustments, the team will shift to high-level medical care that also takes specialty into account.

Organisms that Change Their Shape Adjusting to the Situation

The plasmodium of the slime mould *Physarum polycephalum* is a polynuclear single-celled amoeboid organism consisting of a dendritic network of tube-like structures. Japanese scientist Professor Toshiyuki Nakagaki and his team researched the 'intelligence' of the slime mould and twice received the Ig Nobel Prize for his work.

A representative study involved the slime mould's ability to solve mazes (Nakagaki, Yamada & Tóth, 2000). If the slime mould is spread in a maze box and bait is placed at two spots in the maze, tubes will be created in all paths that gather in the bait, and a liquid called protoplast will enter the tube. Then, as protoplasm flows back and forth in the tube, the liquid gathers in a path that flows easily according to the necessary and unnecessary adaptation rule and becomes thicker and pulls out of the dead-end paths of the maze. Gradually, the long path connecting the two baits narrows and disappears, eventually creating a network that covers the shortest distance necessary to solve the maze.

Another representative study involved the formation of a traffic network by the slime mould (Tero et al., 2010). In this experiment, bait was placed on 30 major cities on the map of the Tokyo metropolitan area in Japan, and slime mould was placed in the centre of Tokyo. The slime mould spread gradually, and when it found food, it left a small body at the feeding place and repeatedly spread to find the next bait. The resultant pattern was very similar to the existing railway network in the Tokyo metropolitan area, from three perspectives: economic efficiency (whether the entire network was the shortest possible), fault tolerance (formation of the circuit) and efficiency of connection between two points. In the real world, it is difficult for all these three factors to be simultaneously optimised, making it necessary to compromise. In other words, the slime mould formed a network by achieving multi-objective optimisation.

Slime moulds share information about food and pathways in the front part of their bodies and adapt their shapes by distributing their resources, even though they do not have central functions such as a brain. Thus, they operate as an autonomous distributed system with cooperativity created by connection.

Slime mould is a single-cell organism, but it behaves as if it were making an incremental decision. This behavioural mechanism for solving complex problems may be more efficient than a deliberated plan and is expected to be applied to new navigation system technology.

Collapsible and Scalable Medical Teams: Medical Teams that Change 'Shape' According to the Situation

Now, we wish to examine the actions of the emergency medical team. First, the emergency medical team called for help to avoid staff shortages and then roughly assigned roles. As patients were transported and evaluated, staff members gradually gathered to deal with severely ill patients, and doctors were reallocated based on their specialties. Notably, although the leader finally permitted, team members changed their roles on their own based on the information exchanged at the bedside, and reallocations were performed through autonomous proposals from each member of the staff. Thus, each team and member were connected, and the size and 'shape' of the teams autonomously changed as information was shared among them, analogous to a slime mould establishing the most efficient network (Figure 5.2). In other words, the autonomous distributed system dynamically and adaptively designed teams and their networks while achieving multi-objective optimisation of medical staff, patient factors and quality of care. A flexible response that adapts to dynamically changing situations is based on multi-objective optimisation, starting with coarse approximation while assuming the worst, and then performing fine adjustment according to the necessary and unnecessary adaptation rule. In particular, after assessing their own medical resources, which were changing dynamically, each team member continuously monitored and repeatedly evaluated the information in front of them (number of patients, severity and condition), and then shared and reallocated the necessary medical resources. It is important to repeat this fine adjustment by iterating the reassessment and reallocation processes.

1. The emergency team first called for help. 2. Staff members were deployed based on a rough assessment. 3. Initial treatment was started by the temporary teams. 4. While proceeding with medical treatment, the team repeatedly reassessed the situations and reallocated resources more appropriately. In reassessment and reallocation, each member acted autonomously based on local information while maintaining connections with other team members. The network was created and dynamically altered by multi-objective optimisation through exchange of information among staff members.

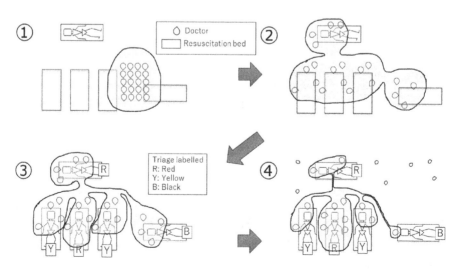

FIGURE 5.2 Adaptive network of the emergency medical team

It can be said that the emergency medical team is obviously making an incremental decision. Both the slime mould and the emergency medical team are making an incremental decision while solving complex problems in a dynamically changing environment, and the essence of this mechanism is to start with coarse approximation, followed by frequent reassessment and reallocation to make fine adjustment.

ROLE OF THE LEADER

The leader plays an important role in the team. In order for the team to make adaptive movements, it is important for team members to move autonomously, but this does not mean that leaders are not necessary. Information from each frontline team member is important, but its scope is necessarily limited to that individual's field of view. Therefore, it is important to take a holistic view from the leader's perspective so that the whole team works towards a common purpose. For example, in this case, the leader asked some doctors who were not otherwise occupied to take photographs. This can be regarded as ensuring adequate backup is available in case the situation deteriorates.

Another role of the leader is the fine adjustment of reallocations made autonomously by team members. The leader was also considering not only the actual events in the emergency room, but also resources outside the emergency department (e.g., the ICU, operating theatre, ambulance and coordination with other medical institutions). In this case, the leader performed cross-boundary coordination between hospital departments and regional hospitals, including management of inpatient beds, including ICU beds, in case the resources in the emergency department became saturated. The leader plays an important role in the team's incremental decision-making as an information network and hub also through coordinating with areas outside of the emergency department.

LEARNING ORGANISATION

Let us now consider why an emergency medical team can achieve such a flexible performance. First, it is useful for medical staff to be aware of how their daily clinical work can be applied to unexpected clinical events. In our emergency department, we hold a bed control meeting with various professionals across related units, including ICU and SDU, every morning and evening and create a bed control plan in case a large number of patients are transferred. Flexible bed control is enabled by repeatedly reviewing the plan according to changes in the situation and executing the plan when the number of patients actually increases. By knowing what we are doing well in daily clinical work, we are able to adapt and respond to unexpected events.

In addition, we hold multidisciplinary joint debriefing sessions, especially in cases that are thought to be highly suggestive from the perspective of disaster response and team approach. Participating staff grasp events from a bird's-eye view, aim to improve team performance while exchanging opinions from the perspective of multiple professions, share opinions about successful points and options, and make efforts to connect to future clinical practice. Although a local incident case like this might occur only once a year or less, the daily multidisciplinary joint meeting and the debriefing sessions were considered useful.

INTERPRETATION

The performance of an emergency medical team responding to an unexpected clinical event is analogous to that of a slime mould, which performs multi-objective optimisation by repeatedly performing complex trade-offs based on available information while maintaining an autonomous distributed system. It also resonates with Lindblom's ideas in his papers on muddling through (Lindblom, 1959, 1979).

The emergency medical team first applied coarse approximations according to their resources and workload. The team then repeatedly reassessed the situations and adjusted resource allocation finely. The study suggested that coarse approximation, frequent reassessment and fine adjustment can be the strategy to be implicitly taken when the medical team muddled through the situation with uncertainty. Even better, multi-objective optimisation balancing medical resources, patient number and severity, and quality of treatment can be achieved over time along with the local information exchange among clinicians, similarly to the way the slime mould finds the most efficient routes to the bait.

CONCLUSION

This case study revealed that the collapsible and scalable emergency medical team, which demonstrated resilient performance in the face of a changing situation by autonomously using limited resources, did not begin through fine adjustment, but instead adapted through coarse approximation, followed by frequent reassessment and reallocation.

REFERENCES

Lindblom, C. E. (1959). The science of "muddling through". *Public Administration Review*, 79–88.
Lindblom, C. E. (1979). Still muddling, not yet through. *Public Administration Review*, 39(6), 517–526.
Nakagaki, T., Yamada, H., & Tóth, Á. (2000). Maze-solving by an amoeboid organism. *Nature*, 407, 470.
Tero, A., Takagi, S., Saigusa, T., Ito, K., Bebber, D. P., Fricker, M. D., … Nakagaki, T. (2010). Rules for biologically inspired adaptive network design. *Science*, 327(5964), 439–442.

6 From Mortality and Morbidity Conference to Quality Assessment Meeting
Step-by-Step Improving Team Resilience

Jaap F. Hamming and Marit S. de Vos

CONTENTS

Innovation in all fields of medicine has brought an increasing opportunity to treat diseases. However, medical care in general and especially surgery harbours an intrinsic risk, which can never be ruled out completely. The results of surgical interventions are not completely predictable and therefore intrinsically unsafe. Some adverse events are foreseeable, for instance, surgical site infections, which can be anticipated and one can try to minimise to a certain extent. But there is always a risk of less foreseeable events. Adverse events can often have a limited impact on the patient's recovery and health, but sometimes lead to serious consequences or even death. Reduction of adverse events has been a long-standing challenge for all surgical specialties and strategies to reduce adverse events have been developed and shared, but progress is slow and surgical groups sometimes struggle. A low number of adverse events has always been seen as an important indicator for quality of surgical care. Over the years surgeons have struggled with the question how to address adverse events and how to learn from them.

THE TRADITIONAL MORTALITY AND MORBIDITY CONFERENCE

For quality assessment in surgery, the focus has traditionally been on adverse events, cases with morbidity and mortality, which are reviewed and discussed in the so-called Mortality and Morbidity (M&M) conferences. The purpose of these meetings is to take a closer view on the circumstances of an adverse event, which has brought harm to the patient. By discussing the case in depth, learning points are retrieved hoping that in the future these events can be avoided and care can be improved. The Accreditation Council for Graduate Medical Education (ACGME) in the US among many others acknowledges the importance of these conferences. As early as 1983, the ACGME demanded all medical specialist training programmes to set up M&M conferences on a regular basis (Accreditation Council for Graduate Medical Education, 1995) and M&M conferences are part of standard practice in many health systems all over the world.

The history of M&M conferences stretches back more than a hundred years with little development of knowledge on how these meetings could be best organised to exploit their full potential. Hence all individual hospital departments muddle through (bi-)weekly case discussions, moving from one conference to the next without a good conceptualisation of why success was not achieved in this particular case, whereas successful outcomes were achieved in all those other (similar) cases. With the growing public interest in the preventability of harm caused by medical interventions, research on improvement of M&M conferences has evolved. Several studies have been published with a general tendency to report positively on the innovations made (Kwok, et al., 2017). Very little is known however on what really contributes to the learning effect, let alone what helps to reduce the number of adverse events, or what improves the quality of care, if that is measurable at all. Similarly, in the Netherlands, case-based discussions of morbidity and mortality are mandatory in the training programmes of medical specialties. The intentions and quality of these meetings are key points in the regular inspection of training programmes and necessary for the accreditation of the training programme. Moreover, M&M conferences are an important part of the quality assessment in the mandatory auditing of surgical departments by the Association of Surgeons of the Netherlands. Here, too, the shared goal of M&M conferences is learning and quality improvement, but to what extent this is achieved is unclear. In general, there appears to be considerable heterogeneity in how M&M meetings are structured, conducted and who is attending (Gore, 2006). A study comparing two very different M&M conferences in a hospital in the US and the Netherlands revealed that similar challenges were encountered in both settings (de Vos, Marang-van de Mheen, Smith, Mou, Whang & Hamming, 2018). Although the survey participants indicated that educational objectives were well met, expectations for quality improvement were not. In another in-depth analysis of the organisation of M&M conferences several barriers and facilitators were identified (de Vos, Hamming & Marang-van de Mheen, 2017). For instance, health care culture, the different hierarchical and expertise levels and the risk of 'shame and blame' can complicate M&M practice, which accentuates the importance of good leadership and role-modelling by senior team members. So, there are organisational and potentially cultural problems with

M&M conferences. Besides, adverse events only represent a small part of the delivered care and learning from everyday clinical work and thus normal practice or good practice is disregarded. The fact that those who have initially designed M&M practice had chosen as an approach to only review cases with adverse outcomes; this can be considered an example of 'muddling through'. Discussing only negative outcomes has since become accepted as the golden standard of meetings for learning and improvement.

THE NEED FOR A NOVEL FORMAT FOR MORTALITY AND MORBIDITY CONFERENCES

Four years ago, the long-standing tradition of the M&M conferences in the Department of Surgery at the Leiden University Medical Center was submitted for a closer look, because of some levels of dissatisfaction with the format and effectivity of the conference among the surgical staff. One of the ambivalent thoughts was that the delivered care shifted from department-based to team-based in the specific fields of surgery. Therefore, a whole surgical department M&M meeting seemed less appropriate and a meeting for specific surgical teams was considered more desirable. There was a clear wish to find a new way, which would meet the needs for learning and quality assessment and improvement. And the focus should be on the collective reflection by the surgical team involved. Because it was not entirely clear what format would be best applicable, the team members of the subspecialties of the Department of Surgery were challenged to explore for themselves what would work best for their surgical service. The desire to reflect on the work performed by teams, instead of individual performance or a whole department, is supported by the literature. As part of a teamwork process, reflection with and by the team can enable them to optimise their potential and performance (Schmutz & Eppich, 2017).

Traditionally, our M&M conferences were weekly meetings with the surgical staff and residents from all surgical services: General, Gastrointestinal, Oncology, Trauma and Transplantation. These weekly meetings were a long-standing tradition for more than 25 years. There was a need for retaining and improving the learning potential and to have more attention directed towards quality improvement. Most professionals work in teams and reflect on their work continuously. The team members of the specialties felt that more specific M&M conferences for the specialties were warranted, so specific subspecialty M&M conferences were installed. Also, there was a strong desire to reflect on, and learn from, cases without the adverse events. This wider perspective would help to learn about why most of the everyday clinical work goes well, and which adaptations were needed to get the job done. The surgeons felt also that administrative compliance issues were insufficiently addressed and needed sorting out. Besides there was an explicit wish to pay attention to the teamwork provided and how this could be improved. Therefore, it was decided that the surgical teams that work together closely address their specific teamwork issues and reflect on them on a regular basis to evaluate the effectiveness of their teamwork together and in relation to other teams.

THE QUALITY ASSESSMENT MEETING

Since 2016 the M&M conference was converted to a weekly Quality Assessment Meeting (QAM) for every surgical specialty service of the Department of Surgery. In addition, the specialties meet for a monthly 'Surgical Academic Conference' to share what has been learned from the specific QAMs. The content of the meetings was revised from a Safety-I (only attention for adverse events), to a Safety-II and resilience perspective (including attention on why things usually go right). The purpose was to monitor outcomes regularly and to learn from daily practice, which includes many patient cases that went well in addition to those that experienced adverse events. The short loop enables learning from things that are still fresh in memory and to make improvements directly on the basis of the case discussions. Furthermore, there was a need to anticipate what could be expected for planned cases. So, patients that were to be admitted for surgical care the following week were now also reviewed for potential risks and to see if certain aspects require extra attention or preparation.

A new format for the QAM was developed and the different surgical specialties applied these principles in the way they considered best with some variations in style and format. The Vascular Surgery Division started with a weekly evaluation of all admitted patients. The QAM is prepared by the attending physician and resident. Administrative aspects such as diagnosis and procedure codes, correspondence to referring physicians, outpatient clinic appointments for follow-up, and registration of adverse events and incidents are checked and corrected or completed when necessary. All cases are reviewed in terms of content of the clinical course, adverse events and lessons to be learned. With equal attention, patients who did well despite anticipated hurdles are discussed, and learning points with special attention to resilient behaviour are brought to QAM members' attention. Also, the communication with the patient and the family is reviewed as well as possible points of improvement in the cooperation between medical and nursing staff. With respect to the main theme of this book: many forms of muddling through-like behaviour come to light in discussions of discharged cases. Moreover, by doing this for all cases, every week, one can reveal patterns of muddling through behaviour that might deserve greater attention, such as recurring problems that constantly require adaptive actions from staff. At first, administrational aspects were reviewed with the whole team, but this took too much time and decreased time available for learning from the clinical course of patients. Thus, in the next phase, administrative aspects were from then on managed by the attendings and reviewed only briefly in the QAM itself, and only discussed when necessary. The grading of adverse event severity (according to a modified Cavien-Dindo classification (Clavien, et al., 2009) is discussed with the whole team, and a specific reflection on whether an event could have been avoided is performed. Other adverse events as well as mortality are discussed and learning points are documented. For the purpose of time management, patients with a brief hospitalisation without specific points of interest (e.g., percutaneous transluminal angioplasties of the peripheral arteries) are given only limited consideration. At this time, endovascularly treated patients are reviewed and discussed in the multidisciplinary meeting with the interventional radiologists, which can be considered as a next step in improving the quality assessment.

Through balancing reflecting on what went wrong with reflecting on what went well, the atmosphere of the meeting has improved compared to the classical M&M conference. Thereby it seems possible to overcome the tempting tendency in classical M&M conferences to glide towards 'blame and shame'. The second part of the meeting consists of looking forward to the patients to be admitted in the next week. The preoperative screening of the anaesthesiologist is reviewed for specific supportive measures needed, extra medication and consultation of relevant other specialties like cardiology and pulmonology. Medication is reviewed with special attention for adjustments of perioperative anticoagulation and thrombocyte aggregation medication, which is always an issue in vascular patients. The surgical plan, which has been previously discussed in a multidisciplinary deliberation, is reviewed and where deemed necessary adjusted. Nowadays a standard format is used to record the anticipated briefing in the electronic medical record, so the considerations of the team are visible for all involved professionals and patients themselves.

THE QAM MEETING TO ADDRESS THE POTENTIALS FOR RESILIENT PERFORMANCE

The design of the QAM allows the surgical team to reflect on their performance in a short feedback loop. Although a formal assessment has not yet been performed, the potentials for resilient performance (learning; anticipating; monitoring; responding) can be found in this set-up (Hollnagel, 2015). The QAM helps the team to monitor what they have done over the past week with patients that were admitted in the hospital and were trusted to their care. Responses to regular and irregular disturbances and to critical issues are reviewed and evaluated. Possible process adjustments are identified and can be implemented swiftly. The weekly meeting enables team learning from cases that went well, as well as from cases with adverse events. Learning points are documented, retrieved regularly and re-discussed.

A typical example is the problems encountered with endovascular access to the arteries of the arm. Endovascular treatment of complex aortic aneurysms necessitates access to the arteries of the arm, besides access to groin arteries. These arteries are more vulnerable and thus more complications are encountered. By regularly reviewing access problems in the arm, we were able to discuss the problems in depth and reflect not only on the improvement of the surgical technique but also to find ways to prevent these problems beforehand.

Anticipation of upcoming inpatient cases has led to improvement of care. Since the introduction of the QAM no more patients have dropped out of the theatre schedule because of insufficient preparations for surgery. Also, last moment adjustments of admitted patients have been reduced, which in turn reduces the variability in care and creates a more stable admittance process. As such, the QAM in this novel format has already served an important need – to enhance the resilience of the surgical team. The team has been able to implement a true on-the-spot team reflection, which can be documented in the patient file, and thereby is transparent for all involved professionals and patients. We have experienced an enhanced feeling of team spirit and improvement in teamwork.

FUTURE IMPROVEMENTS

Further improvements to the QAM format are pressing and require attention. Until recently, the input of the nursing staff in the QAM has been insufficient. Points of attention were collected from the nursing staff on a regular basis, especially in the preparation of the meeting itself. But in the first years the nurses only rarely participated in the QAM for logistical and scheduling reasons. When they did participate, they commented that the discussions were too focussed on medical issues and less on matters of importance to nursing. Nowadays the nurses do participate in the QAM: they retrieve relevant issues for specific patients from their colleagues and attend the meeting when we review the past cases. They comment on the reflections by the physicians and supplement the reflections by specific concerns of the nurses. So, another step forward has been made.

Another important desire is to have multidisciplinary discussions for instance between surgeons and anaesthesiologists or intensivists. Logistic factors such as finding an agreed time to meet have hampered further implementation and improvement. A specifically tedious and frustrating subject is the accessibility of the electronic medical record file (EMR) for quality assessment. The structure of data filing in the EMR is such that it is not well equipped for data analysis at this time. Improvements are urgently needed, but unfortunately very dependent on the willingness of the EMR production companies and budget. In a QAM, the lessons learned primarily apply to those attending that specific meeting. What can we do to retain these lessons for the team members that were not able to attend the meeting or for future team members? At this time, there is not yet a system in place to archive lessons from cases that went well, which can be used to document how the team adapted to the expected and unexpected clinical situations. Currently, we are designing a system in which it is possible to store the lessons. In a designated QAM these lessons can be retrieved and reflected on, in an attempt to store these lessons in the division's 'collective memory'.

The surgical QAM serves the need to reflect on the care that is actually delivered by the surgical team and to anticipate on what can be expected for the scheduled inpatient cases. This format enhances the resilience of our surgical teams and addresses the four cornerstones of resilience engineering. Our surgical divisions are going to a next phase of learning from each other to improve the meetings, and to find ways to extend the team resilience to other clinical departments and professional teams. Every surgical or medical (sub)specialty is different and has its own specific logistic demands, which makes a 'one size fits all' approach impossible. However, the principles to achieve resilience are similar and every department and team has to explore ways to accomplish a QAM of their own. A critical issue is that the teams have to find the time and opportunity to hold discussions on their delivered care – to understand everyday clinical work which will bring a rich harvest of knowledge – and to anticipate the near future.

REFERENCES

Accreditation Council for Graduate Medical Education. (1995). Essentials and information items. In G. Gupta (Ed.), *Graduate Medical Education Directory, 1995–1996*. Chicago, IL: American Medical Association.

Clavien, P. A., Barkun, J., de Oliveira, M. L., Vauthey, J. N., Dindo, D., Schulick, R. D., … Makuuchi, M. (2009). The Clavien-Dindo classification of surgical complications: Five-year experience. *Annals of Surgery*, 250(2), 187–196.

de Vos, M. S., Hamming, J. F., & Marang-van de Mheen, P. J. (2017). Barriers and facilitators to learn and improve through morbidity and mortality conferences: A qualitative study. *BMJ Open*, 7, e01883.

de Vos, M. S., Marang-van de Mheen, P. J., Smith, A. D., Mou, D., Whang, E. E., & Hamming, J. F. (2018). Toward best practices for surgical morbidity and mortality conferences: A mixed methods study. *Journal of Surgical Education*, 75(1), 33–42.

Gore, D. C. (2006). National survey of surgical morbidity and mortality conferences. *American Journal of Surgery*, 191(5), 708–714.

Hollnagel, E. (2015). *Introduction to the Resilience Analysis Grid (RAG)*. Retrieved 30 August 2019, from http://erikhollnagel.com/onewebmedia/RAG Outline V2.pdf.

Kwok, E. S. H., Calder, L. A., Barlow-Krelina, E., Mackie, C., Seely, A. J. E., Cwinn, R., … Frank, J. R. (2017). Implementation of a structured hospital-wide morbidity and mortality rounds model. *BMJ Quality and Safety*, 26(6), 439–448.

Schmutz, J. B., & Eppich, W. J. (2017). Promoting learning and patient care through shared reflection: A conceptual framework for team reflexivity in health care. *Academic Medicine*, 92(11), 1555–1563.

7 Images of Work-as-Imagined

Jennifer Jackson

CONTENTS

INTRODUCTION

There is much discussion of the gap between Work-as-Imagined and Work-as-Done in the health care context, with various authors suggesting closing, or otherwise addressing, this gap. Work-as-Imagined is the work that is anticipated, under normal conditions. Work-as-Done, in contrast, is what actually happens in complex contexts (Hollnagel, Wears, & Braithwaite, 2015). While there is extensive research exploring the concept of Work-as-Done, the ways in which Work-as-Imagined has been explored are limited. The definition of Work-as-Imagined implies more than policy, yet it is almost exclusively represented in the literature as written policies and protocols.

In its manifestation as policies and protocols, Work-as-Imagined has primarily been understood in terms of how it relates to Work-as-Done. This is reflected in publications that emphasise the gap between Work-as-Imagined and Work-as-Done, and the ways in which planned work differs from enacted work (Anderson et al., 2019a; Anderson, Ross, Back, Duncan, & Jaye, 2019b; Anderson et al., 2016; Back et al., 2017; Clay-Williams, Hounsgaard, & Hollnagel, 2015; Damen et al., 2018; Hannigan, Simpson, Coffey, Barlow, & Jones, 2018; Nakajima, 2015; Nakajima, Masuda, & Nakajima, 2017). Such works detail different aspects of the gap, with recommendations to improve training, create flexible policies, and increased support for staff. Most studies describe the nature of the gap between Work-as-Imagined and Work-as-Done (Anderson, Ross, & Jaye, 2017; Johnson & Lane, 2017; McNab, Bowie, Morrison, & Ross, 2016), with some exploring factors that perpetuate the gap (Hollnagel, 2015; Hunte & Wears, 2017). In contrast, others focus on how this gap may be closed (Clay-Williams & Braithwaite, 2017; Patterson, Deutsch, & Jacobson, 2017; Wears & Hunte, 2017). These studies argue that if the system is designed appropriately, Work-as-Imagined should be the same as Work-as-Done. Others do not agree that alignment is possible, or that it would necessarily produce better outcomes (Anderson et al., 2016).

Efforts to reconcile Work-as-Imagined and Work-as-Done have shown that this process is more complex than simply amending policy. In a health care context, it is inevitable that everyday clinical work will present continuous challenges and problems. Nursing work, for example, is complex (Ebright, 2010; Ebright, Patterson, Chalko, & Render, 2003) and often requires tacit knowledge (Herbig, Bussing, & Ewert, 2001) to make on-the-spot decisions. An understanding of Work-as-Imagined that goes beyond written policies and protocols can identify what factors may drive the response to unexpected conditions.

This chapter presents a part of a larger study that examined the nature of nursing work through the lens of resilient health care. This chapter explores Work-as-Imagined for nurses, to determine how comprehensively it is captured by written policies, what other forms of the concept may be influential in clinical work, and how nurses navigate – or muddle through with purpose – everyday clinical work in the context of their Work-as-Imagined.

METHODS

Nurses across the United Kingdom were invited to participate in this study and were recruited through social media, email lists, and word of mouth. These nurses work in a variety of settings, including community care and mental health. Participants played a scenario-based serious video game *Resilience Challenge* (Jackson et al., 2020) where participants made choices to guide a patient's journey through the hospital. This game was part of a semi-structured interview about nurses' everyday clinical work. While playing the game, participants explained their priorities in each scenario to the researcher, and how they would respond to less than ideal circumstances. Each of these scenarios required a degree of muddling through, as the options available to participants required compromises. Interviews lasted 45–150 minutes and were audio recorded and transcribed verbatim.

The analysis technique in this study was interpretive description (Thorne, 2008; Thorne, Kirkham, & MacDonald-Emes, 1997; Thorne, Kirkham, & O'Flynn-Magee, 2004). Interview transcripts were analysed to identify concepts and interpret how participants understood and responded to these concepts. The analysis focussed on examples of what nurses drew on to inform their process of muddling through in challenging circumstances. It became apparent there was more than one aspect of Work-as-Imagined influencing nurses' everyday clinical work. These findings are presented in detail in the following section.

FINDINGS

The demographic profiles of participants in this study are summarised in Table 7.1. There were 20 participants in total: 16 female participants and 4 male participants.

TABLE 7.1

Demographic profiles of participants

Characteristic	No of Participants	%
Age		
20–29 years	5	25
30–39 years	8	40
40–49 years	6	30
50–59 years	1	5
Level of Education		
Student	4	20
Bachelor	5	25
Masters	8	40
PhD	3	15
Ethnicity		
White – British	15	75
White – European	4	20
Black – Caribbean	1	5
Total Years of Work Experience		
Less than 5	4	20
5–9	4	20
10–14	4	20
15–19	4	20
20+	4	20
Domain of Nursing		
Adult	16	80
Mental health	2	10
Child	1	5
Learning disability	1	5

The participants represent a mix of ages, experience and education. The majority practice in adult nursing and identify as white British. These participants work in a variety of settings, including community-based care, which is an addition to the resilient health care research that involves largely hospital-based staff.

The findings of the current study indicated that there are multiple types of Work-as-Imagined. While written policies and guidelines are fundamental elements, other factors also constitute Work-as-Imagined. These other types of Work-as-Imagined were named external-formal, external-informal, and internal (relative to the person doing the work). These categories are not clear cut, and the lines between them blur in practice. Each of these is discussed in the following sections.

EXTERNAL-FORMAL WORK-AS-IMAGINED

External-formal types of Work-as-Imagined are formalised documents that provide direct guidance for clinical work. These include legal requirements, policies, and evidence. Nurses were quick to identify these elements as part of their work. Legal requirements form the foundational standards for nurses, providing the fundamental guidelines for their work. Even when under pressure, the nurses who participated in this study reported they were careful to observe legal requirements. For example, nurses in mental health settings reported that the Mental Health Act was a reference point when patients were required to stay in hospital, recognising that if they failed to follow the letter of the law in such cases, they could be detaining the patient illegally. Therefore, they adhered strictly to this legislation in all circumstances. Legal documents were seen as a tool of satisficing; that is, providing the basic minimum standard for care.

Written policies and protocols, as expected, form part of nurses' Work-as-Imagined. Nurses reported that they use these types of Work-as-Imagined to direct their practice, even though they are limited in some areas. For example, one advanced nurse practitioner reported that though her scope of practice could be expanded, a policy had not been revised to allow her to work to her full capacity. Her colleagues who were required to change the policy prioritised their clinical work over updating documents. In turn, this advanced nurse practitioner's practice was restricted because the policy was not in place to enable her to work to her full scope. Other participants reported similar experiences, outlining the difficulties they had encountered when it came to updating policies and merging legal requirements with the realities of clinical work.

Other nurses recognised that they should use policies as a foundation of their work, but found that certain policies made this impossible. In these cases, Work-as-Imagined could not be aligned with Work-as-Done, and nurses were required to muddle through with purpose. For example, a participant explained that policies were written with the assumption that the patient would be white, English speaking, a British citizen and securely housed, among other things. However, many patients are undocumented, do not speak English, use substances, and experience homelessness. In such cases, nurses said they were unable to use policies to guide their work, because policies are created for a 'model patient'. The appropriate adaptive actions for patients who required modifications were not prescribed in guiding documents. The requirements of vulnerable patients were not represented in written policies, and thus the policies were set aside in favour of experiential clinical strategies. Nurses were required to muddle through with purpose, because of the lack of appropriate guidelines. Some participants reported that they enjoyed this process, because muddling was an opportunity to be creative and connect with others. Nurses also gained satisfaction from knowing they had overcome limitations to help vulnerable people.

Research evidence constituted another external-formal aspect of Work-as-Imagined. Such evidence was particularly important for those nurses who worked with specific populations and kept up to date with publications in a key area. For example, a study might demonstrate the efficacy of a new medication, but when the inclusion/exclusion criteria for the study were restricted (i.e., had taken no medication previously), many patients fell outside the research parameters. These patients with complex chronic illnesses were rarely involved in clinical trials and had moved beyond available evidence or practice guidelines. In these cases, the nurse had to muddle through by working with colleagues to try and incrementally adjust medication ad hoc, because there was no suitable source of guidance.

These external-formal types of Work-as-Imagined were well represented in participant responses in the current study. The limitations in external-formal Work-as-Imagined required nurses to muddle through with purpose, because there may have been limited sources of information to guide their work. This has the potential to create additional burden for nurses, when they are required to adapt their work on the spot.

Participants also reported other types of Work-as-Imagined, which have not previously been documented. These are external-informal, and internal, and are discussed in the following sections.

EXTERNAL-INFORMAL SOURCES OF WORK-AS-IMAGINED

One of the most influential external-informal forms of Work-as-Imagined for participants in the current study were workplace norms and culture. Much of their clinical work was based on the idea of 'that's how we do things/have always done things here'. Some routines, such as how and when patients were washed, illustrate the ways in which ward norms operated. Several participants discussed the way wards' bathing routines were socially enforced, even if the patient did not need or want to be washed. These informal expectations of clinical practice could create extra work; for example, nurses were expected to change their work for each physician, to match the physician's preferences. These types of workplace norms were not overtly questioned, because nurses did not feel they had the social capital to change the local culture, or because they feared retribution. However, there was also an opportunity to achieve excellence, when nurses were empowered to overcome challenges through their work. The workplace culture was very influential and could support high standards in nurses' work.

Patient expectations represent another type of external-informal Work-as-Imagined. Nurses reported that they aimed to meet the needs of patients, often collaborating with them in ways that made their nursing work rewarding. In some cases, however, nurses felt that patients' expectations were unrealistic. For example, a participant described the 'Amazon Culture' of an emergency department, where patients would arrive requesting urgent tests, and leave before the results were reported. This participant explained that the idea of receiving packages almost immediately from the retailer Amazon influenced this patient's expectations of health care services. Other such instances involved patients requesting new medications or procedures that had yet to be approved. Patients arrived for care with their own versions of Work-as-Imagined, which nurses could find difficult to manage when they were at odds with the realities of everyday clinical work.

INTERNAL SOURCES OF WORK-AS-IMAGINED

Nurses also identified their internal ideas about being a nurse as a source of Work-as-Imagined. For instance, several nurses reported that they wanted to spend time providing emotional support to patients. However, as the pressures of their work environment made the giving of such support difficult, many felt they had failed to be a 'good nurse'. In some cases, these internal standards had a negative impact, with nurses skipping breaks or staying extra hours to finish their work. One participant reflected on images of nurses as saintly women, saying she felt pressure to meet that standard (or that of Florence Nightingale). These internalised ideas of who was a 'good nurse' were significant for participants and were the benchmark nurses used to evaluate their performance. Nurses also used their internal ideas of being a good nurse as supporting their work, as they avoided satisficing in favour of upholding their high standards.

Some nurses felt ashamed if their work fell short of that ideal. Nurses reported feeling this way, even though their work exists in a complex system. The non-linearity of outcomes indicates that nurses felt responsible (or were held accountable) for outcomes they could not necessarily have predicted. Internal sources of Work-as-Imagined could also create conflict, because nurses would inevitably have personal versions of 'good nursing' that could be at odds with their colleagues' ideas.

The other main aspect of internal Work-as-Imagined was lessons from experience. Nurses used their personal experiences to inform their care, and reported learning from situations where things went well. For example, participants explained how they could imagine the care plan just by looking at a patient. Experience developed over the course of nurses' careers, and informed their expectations about likely scenarios they would encounter. Therefore, new nurses were less able to draw on this source of Work-as-Imagined to inform their work, relative to experienced colleagues.

Each of these types of Work-as-Imagined influences how nurses do their work, in different ways. These findings demonstrate that the factors driving ideas of how work should be done are more complex than written policies or protocols (Table 7.2). As a result, it can be difficult to identify the precise cause of the gap between Work-as-Imagined and Work-as-Done.

These findings demonstrate that the properties of Work-as-Imagined are more complex than previously thought. Participants used external-formal sources of Work-as-Imagined in the form of written policies and protocols, as it is commonly understood. However, nurses also identified external-informal and internal sources of Work-as-Imagined that formed their working idea of what nurses do. These findings are important when exploring why nurses need to muddle through with purpose, which is discussed in the following section.

TABLE 7.2
Types of Work-as-Imagined

Type of Work-as-Imagined	Example
External-formal	Written policies and protocols
	Legal guidelines
	Evidence
External-informal	Workplace norms and culture
	Patient expectations
Internal	Personal ideals of being a 'good nurse'
	Experience

DISCUSSION

The definition of Work-as-Imagined as what will happen under anticipated normal working conditions (Hollnagel et al., 2015) is supported by this study. Work-as-Imagined has been characterised as formal guidance on how to work, such as that provided by written policies and protocols (Anderson Ross, Back, Duncan, & Jaye et al., 2019b; Anderson et al., 2016). This study adds that Work-as-Imagined is broader than written policies and protocols, as policies do not capture the full range of expectations of how work happens. External-informal and internal sources of Work-as-Imagined should also be considered when examining everyday clinical work.

External-informal sources of Work-as-Imagined have a documented impact on outcomes. For participants, workplace norms dictated the informal standards of their work, creating a type of Work-as-Imagined. In one study, nurses attributed their theory-practice gap to their workplace conditions (Maben, Latter, & Macleod, 2006). Similarly, Aiken et al. (2011) have shown that nurses require a good work environment to provide quality care and decrease mortality rates. When a health care environment is constrained, staff must provide care in a context of 'organisational sabotage' (Maben et al., 2006, p. 469). Organisational sabotage occurred when nurses had the intention to provide exemplary care, but organisational pressures like limited staffing or excessive workload prevented nurses from working to their standards.

Nurses' internal standards and their experience represent another type of Work-as-Imagined. Nurses in the current study reported that when they could not meet their personal standards, they felt there were negative impacts for themselves as well as their patients. This finding is broadly supported by other research. For example, when nurses felt unable to meet their personal standards, it was a source of considerable guilt and shame (Maben et al., 2006). Health care professionals can experience profound regret, and remember instances where they feel they failed their patients (von Arx et al., 2018; Wolf & Zuzelo, 2006). There is also the potential for nurses to experience moral distress if their ideals of the right kind of care are at odds with workplace norms (Morley, Ives, Bradbury-Jones, & Irvine, 2017). The impact of internal ideas of what work should be is substantial, and should thus be considered an integral part of the concept of Work-as-Imagined.

There are also potential benefits from using Work-as-Imagined to inform muddling through with purpose. Nurses are powerful patient advocates (Bu & Jezewski, 2007), who are willing to engage in muddling through with purpose in order to achieve positive outcomes with patients. The ability to adapt work is part of the art of nursing (Finfgeld-Connett, 2008). Muddling through with purpose could include activities from everyday clinical work to making system-level changes, through political action (Morley & Jackson, 2017). Nurses can be supported to make positive on-the-spot decisions and create better patient outcomes by doing so.

CONCLUSION

Ideas of what should happen under normal conditions (Hollnagel, 2015) go beyond formal documentation of procedures. From these findings, it is clear that Work-as-Imagined, in all its forms, influences how work gets done. For nurses, muddling through with purpose is a way of dealing with Work-as-Imagined in order to get things done in everyday clinical work. This enables resilient health care, but it can also be a source of considerable conflict and moral distress when things do not go as planned. Researchers who want to 'close the gap' between Work-as-Imagined and Work-as-Done would be well served by identifying what type of Work-as-Imagined is influential, rather than assuming that written policies and protocols are the main idea of preferred performance. Changing a health care policy may not result in clinical changes if factors like routines or workplace culture are driving behaviour. Muddling through with purpose occurs in the gap between Work-as-Imagined and Work-as-Done, with the potential for both positive and negative outcomes.

Researchers could identify which type of Work-as-Imagined is most influential in a specific clinical situation and focus on that area to influence Work-as-Done.

REFERENCES

Aiken, L. H., Cimiotti, J. P., Sloane, D. M., Smith, H. L., Flynn, L., & Neff, D. F. (2011). Effects of nurse staffing and nurse education on patient deaths in hospitals with different nurse work environments. *Medical Care*, 49(12), 1047–1053.

Anderson, J. E., Ross, A., Back, J., Duncan, M., Hopper, A., Snell, P., & Jaye, P. (2019a). Resilience engineering for quality improvement. In E. Hollnagel, J. Braithwaite, & R. Wears (Eds.), *Resilient Health Care, Volume 4: Delivering Resilient Health Care* (pp. 32–41). Abingdon, UK: Routledge.

Anderson, J. E., Ross, A., Back, J., Duncan, M., & Jaye, P. (2019b). Resilience engineering as a quality improvement method in healthcare. In S. Wiig & B. Fahlbruch (Eds.), *Exploring Resilience – A Scientific Journey from Practice to Theory* (pp. 25–31). Cham, Switzerland: Springer.

Anderson, J. E., Ross, A., & Jaye, P. (2017). Modelling resilience and researching the gap between Work-as-Imagined and Work-as-Done. In J. Braithwaite, R. Wears, & E. Hollnagel (Eds.), *Resilient Health Care, Volume 3: Reconciling Work-as-Imagined and Work-as-Done* (pp. 133–142). Boca Raton, FL: CRC Press.

Anderson, J. E., Ross, A. J., Back, J., Duncan, M., Snell, P., Walsh, K., & Jaye, P. (2016). Implementing resilience engineering for healthcare quality improvement using the CARE model: A feasibility study protocol. *Pilot and Feasibility Studies*, 2(1), 61–70.

Back, J., Ross, A. J., Duncan, M. D., Jaye, P., Henderson, K., & Anderson, J. E. (2017). Emergency department escalation in theory and practice: A mixed-methods study using a model of organizational resilience. *Annals of Internal Medicine*, 70(5), 659–671.

Bu, X., & Jezewski, M. A. (2007). Developing a mid-range theory of patient advocacy through concept analysis. *Journal of Advanced Nursing*, 57(1), 101–110.

Clay-Williams, R., & Braithwaite, J. (2017). Realigning Work-as-Imagined and Work-as-Done: Can training help? In J. Braithwaite, R. Wears, & E. Hollnagel (Eds.), *Resilient Health Care, Volume 3: Reconciling Work-as-imagined and Work-as-Done* (pp. 153–162). Boca Raton, FL: CRC Press.

Clay-Williams, R., Hounsgaard, J., & Hollnagel, E. (2015). Where the rubber meets the road: Using FRAM to align Work-as-Imagined with Work-as-Done when implementing clinical guidelines. *Implementation Science*, 10, 1–8.

Damen, N. L., de Vos, M. S., Moesker, M. J., Braithwaite, J., de Lind van Wijngaarden, R. A. F., Kaplan, J., … Clay-Williams, R. (2018). Preoperative anticoagulation management in everyday clinical practice: An international comparative analysis of Work-as-Done using the Functional Resonance Analysis Method. *Journal of Patient Safety*. [Epublication ahead of print]. 10.1097/pts.0000000000000515.

Ebright, P. R. (2010). The complex work of RNs: Implications for healthy work environments. *Online Journal of Issues in Nursing*, 15(1).

Ebright, P. R., Patterson, E. S., Chalko, B. A., & Render, M. L. (2003). Understanding the complexity of Registered Nurse work in acute care settings. *Journal of Nursing Administration*, 33(12), 630–638.

Finfgeld-Connett, D. (2008). Concept synthesis of the art of nursing. *Journal of Advanced Nursing*, 62(3), 381–388.

Hannigan, B., Simpson, A., Coffey, M., Barlow, S., & Jones, A. (2018). Care coordination as imagined, care coordination as done: Findings from a cross-national mental health systems study. *International Journal of Integrated Care*, 18(3), 12.

Herbig, B., Bussing, A., & Ewert, T. (2001). The role of tacit knowledge in the work context of nursing. *Journal of Advanced Nursing*, 34(5), 687–695.

Hollnagel, E. (2015). Why is Work-as-Imagined different from Work-as-Done? In R. Wears, E. Hollnagel, & J. Braithwaite (Eds.), *Resilient Health Care, Volume 2: The Resilience of Everyday Clinical Work* (pp. 249–264). Farnham, UK: Ashgate Publishing.

Hollnagel, E., Wears, R. L., & Braithwaite, J. (2015). *From Safety-1 to Safety-2: A White Paper*. Retrieved 4 September 2020, from https://www.england.nhs.uk/signuptosafety/wp-content/uploads/sites/16/2015/10/safety-1-safety-2-whte-papr.pdf.

Hunte, G. S., & Wears, R. (2017). Power and resilience in practice: Fitting a 'square peg in a round hole' in everyday clinical work. In J. Braithwaite, R. Wears, & E. Hollnagel (Eds.), *Resilient Health Care, Volume 3: Reconciling Work-as-Imagined and Work-as-Done* (pp. 119–132). Boca Raton, FL: CRC Press.

Jackson, J., Iacovides, J., Duncan, M., Alders, M., Maben, J., & Anderson, J. (2020). Operationalizing resilient healthcare concepts through a serious video game for clinicians. *Applied Ergonomics*, 87, 103112.

Johnson, A., & Lane, P. (2017). Resilience Work-as-Done in everyday clinical work. In J. Braithwaite, R. Wears, & E. Hollnagel (Eds.), *Resilient Health Care, Volume 3: Reconciling Work-as-Imagined and Work-as-Done* (pp. 71–88). Boca Raton, FL: CRC Press.

Maben, J., Latter, S., & Macleod, J. (2006). The thory – practice gap: Impact of professional – bureaucratic work conflict on newly-qualified nurses. *Journal of Advanced Nursing*, 55(4), 465–477.

McNab, D., Bowie, P., Morrison, J., & Ross, A. (2016). Understanding patient safety performance and educational needs using the 'Safety-II' approach for complex systems. *Education for Primary Care*, 27(6), 443–450.

Morley, G., Ives, J., Bradbury-Jones, C., & Irvine, F. (2017). What is 'moral distress'? A narrative synthesis of the literature. *Nursing Ethics*, 26(3), 646–662.

Morley, G., & Jackson, J. (2017). Is the art of nursing dying? A call for political action. *Journal of Research in Nursing*, 22(5), 342–351.

Nakajima, K. (2015). Blood transfusions with health information technology in emergency settings from a safety-II perspective. In R. Wears, E. Hollnagel, & J. Braithwaite (Eds.), *Resilient Health Care, Volume 2: The Resilience of Everyday Clinical Work* (pp. 99–114). Farnham, UK: Ashgate Publishing.

Nakajima, K., Masuda, S., & Nakajima, S. (2017). Exploring ways to capture and facilitate Work-as-Done that interact with health information technology. In J. Braithwaite, R. Wears, & E. Hollnagel (Eds.), *Resilient Health Care, Volume 3: Reconciling Work-as-Imagined and Work-as-Done* (pp. 61–70). Boca Raton, FL: CRC Press.

Patterson, M., Deutsch, E. S., & Jacobson, L. (2017). Simulation: Closing the gap between Work-as-Imagined and Work-as-Done. In J. Braithwaite, R. Wears, & E. Hollnagel (Eds.), *Resilient Health Care, Volume 3: Reconciling Work-as-Imagined and Work-as-Done* (pp. 143–152). Boca Raton, FL: CRC Press.

Thorne, S. (2008). *Interpretive Description*. Walnut Creek, CA: Left Coast Press.

Thorne, S., Kirkham, S. R., & MacDonald-Emes, J. (1997). Interpretive description: A noncat-
    egorical qualitative alternative for developing nursing knowledge. *Research in Nursing
    and Health*, 20(2), 169–177.
Thorne, S., Kirkham, S. R., & O'Flynn-Magee, K. (2004). The analytic challenge in interpre-
    tive description. *International Journal of Qualitative Methods*, 3(1), 1–11.
von Arx, M., Cullati, S., Schmidt, R. E., Richner, S., Kraehenmann, R., Cheval, B., …
    Courvoisier, D. S. (2018). "We won't retire without skeletons in the closet": Healthcare-
    related regrets among physicians and nurses in German-Speaking Swiss hospitals.
    Qualitative Health Research, 28(11), 1746–1758.
Wears, R., & Hunte, G. S. (2017). Resilient procedures: Oxymoron or innovation? In
    J. Braithwaite, R. Wears, & E. Hollnagel (Eds.), *Resilient Health Care, Volume 3:
    Reconciling Work-as-Imagined and Work-as-Done* (pp. 163–170). Boca Raton, FL:
    CRC Press.
Wolf, Z. R., & Zuzelo, P. R. (2006). "Never Again" stories of nurses: Dilemmas in nursing
    practice. *Qualitative Health Research*, 16(9), 1191–1206.

Part III

The Functional Resonance Analysis Method (FRAM) as a Gateway into Muddling with a Purpose

THE FUNCTIONAL RESONANCE ANALYSIS METHOD (FRAM) AS A GATEWAY INTO MUDDLING WITH A PURPOSE

The Functional Resonance Analysis Method (FRAM) is increasingly used to examine and model the variability of work. It helps people using it to look at how behaviour varies, adapts and alters over time. The four contributions in Part III all use FRAM as their tool of choice to understand muddling-type behaviours.

This section of the book begins with Damen and de Vos who examine their past work in using FRAM in hospitals in the Netherlands. They outline some of the key strengths of FRAM including how it provides insights into Work-as-Done, is readily understood by clinicians, nurses and allied health professionals and is often a good investment in time. As to challenges, key to successful use of FRAM for Damen and de Vos is to practise with it, but to also understand the underlying theory on which it is based.

Moving to Australia, Buikstra, Clay-Williams and Strivens look at an application of FRAM in a ward caring for older people, specifically examining the shift from care on the ward through the discharge planning activities. They applied resilience thinking to their tasks, not only using the FRAM to model their patients' journeys but also applying efficiency – thoroughness trade-off (ETTO) ideas to understand how staff make decisions, balance options and make progress.

Sujan, a regular contributor to the Resilient Health Care volumes, investigates intensive care units and muddling behaviours in medication ordering and management, applying the FRAM to understand Work-as-Done in his research in the United Kingdom. A key finding, mirroring that of Buikstra et al., is that we need to do further work to support and strengthen frontline clinicians' capacity to make trade-offs over time.

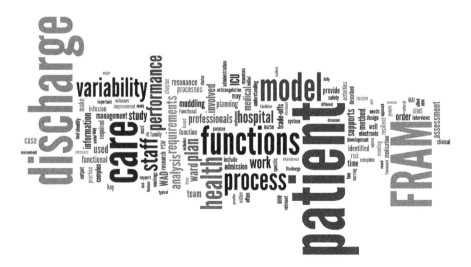

FIGURE 1   A word cloud of Part III. (Source: http://www.wordle.net/)

The final contribution in this section is made by Ransolin, Saurin and Formoso, who adopted FRAM to model connections between patient safety and well-being and its relationship to the built environment. Focussing on the intensive care unit as their object of study, in their FRAM they gathered data via interviews, observations and analysis of regulations, with 85 hours of interviews and ethnographic encounters. This Brazilian research advocates the use of FRAM for a new application – for understanding how the built environment may or may not have important effects on patient safety and well-being (Figure 1).

8 Experiences with FRAM in Dutch Hospitals
Muddling Through with Models

Nikki L. Damen and Marit S. de Vos

CONTENTS

> FRAM offered us a completely new perspective on our anticoagulation management; for years a 'headache file'. We simply never looked at it this way before. Instead of mainly focusing on whether or not we followed the guidelines, we now discussed the process from a daily practice point of view. By doing so, we were able to come up with improvement initiatives that actually improved our work process.
>
> **(Cardiothoracic surgeon)**

Safety-II offers a very promising and welcome new perspective on quality and safety, but it remains a great challenge as to how hospitals can translate this theory into specific research plans and improvement initiatives. We reviewed the Functional

Resonance Analysis Method (FRAM) to visualise and analyse complex processes as they occur in everyday clinical practice. This tool seemed exactly what we were looking for as it provides a practical means to apply Safety-II principles in patient safety work in hospitals.

Since 2017, we conducted FRAM analyses on various health care topics, such as preoperative anticoagulation management (Damen, et al., 2018), critical results in radiology, postpartum haemorrhage, thrombosis prophylaxis, and the triage process at the Emergency Department. All applied FRAM analyses revealed valuable insights into Work-as-Done which provided the base for further process optimisation. In this chapter, we will elaborate on our experiences and provide some recommendations for the practical implementation of FRAM. In addition, we suggest a practical framework to structure the interpretation of the results of a FRAM analysis, to help gain a better understanding of the intricacies of everyday work carried out by health care professionals.

APPLICATIONS OF FRAM

FRAM can be applied for various purposes in the hospital or broader health care setting, such as:

- *Process optimisation*: often this concerns the so-called 'headache files'; complex, multidisciplinary processes where traditional improvement initiatives appeared to be insufficient. This was nicely illustrated by recent studies on transitional care following hospital discharge and sepsis detection combining perspectives from the various professionals involved (O'Hara, Baxter & Hardicre, 2020; Raben, et al., 2018);
- *Incident investigations*: FRAM could also be used as a support tool for incident analysis as it allows studying how an event (a specific 'instantiation' or scenario within the FRAM model) emerged in relation to Work-as-Done rather than only comparing such events with expectations of a process (e.g., protocols). Information on how work normally goes well can then be used to understand why things sometimes go wrong;
- *Guideline development and implementation*: information on Work-as-Done aids critical assessment of available guidelines in relation to real everyday practice, revealing how it may not always be feasible to implement certain steps. Vice versa, FRAM can be used to foster guideline implementation, as insight into Work-as-Done reveals strengths as well as points of concern in the implementation phase, enhancing successful implementation. This was shown in a prior study by Clay-Williams et al. (Clay-Williams, Hounsgaard & Hollnagel, 2015);
- *Intervention development and implementation:* similar to guideline development and implementation, information on Work-as-Done aids understanding of how an intervention is carried out at the actual workplace post-implementation. Based on this, strengths and weaknesses can be identified, providing the base for further improvement. Also, when designing an intervention, it will be

helpful to know Work-as-Done beforehand, enhancing the chance of successful implementation (in an attempt to reconcile Work-as-Imagined and Work-as-Done, as described in previous books);

- *Prospective risk management*: when the Emergency Department of one hospital location merged with that of another location, we made a FRAM analysis on the triage process to examine strengths and risks of the current triage process. These findings provided the base for the design of the triage flow in the new setting.

WHERE TO START?

When introduced to the FRAM theory and the FRAM models for the first time, an often-heard question is 'it looks impressive, but is it not very complex and time-consuming?' This was also our first impression, but once you have muddled through your first analysis, you are confident to take on the next. The FRAM handbook (Hollnagel, Hounsgaard & Colligan, 2014) and website (http://functional-resonance.com) explain the basic principles of the method. Another useful reference on FRAM is the Master Thesis by Jeanette Hounsgaard (Hounsgaard, 2016). In the following paragraphs, we will elaborate on the phases of building the FRAM model and using the definitive model as a tool for discussion with involved professionals.

MODELLING WORK-AS-IMAGINED AND WORK-AS-DONE

In a FRAM model, the main process steps or activities are illustrated in hexagons. The lines between the hexagons reflect interactions and dependencies between activities and hence between the various involved professionals. FRAM provides a useful means to visualise Work-as-Imagined as well as Work-as-Done, triggering a discussion on how to reconcile the two. As the starting point for a FRAM analysis, a model of Work-as-Imagined can be used to visualise what is expected of the process according to (inter)national or local guidelines, protocols and task descriptions. Second, semi-structured interviews with involved frontline professionals can be conducted to obtain insight into Work-as-Done. Having finished the Work-as-Imagined model helps to understand the scope and focus of the interviews, but should not lead to suggestive questions such as whether the professional uses certain protocols. Local observations can also be used to obtain information on how the work is actually carried out. Based on this input, a Work-as-Done FRAM model is made, visualising the process as it is conducted in daily practice. This can be done in an iterative process, in which the model is extended after each interview or observation. In addition to the visual model, it is useful to write a narrative text on how the process is carried out (Hounsgaard, 2016). Figures 8.1, 8.2 and 8.3 show examples of FRAM models on preoperative anticoagulation management for thoracic surgery patients; Figure 8.1 shows an example of a Work-as-Imagined and Figures 8.2 and 8.3 are of Work-as-Done in Australian and Dutch hospitals, respectively (Damen et al., 2018).

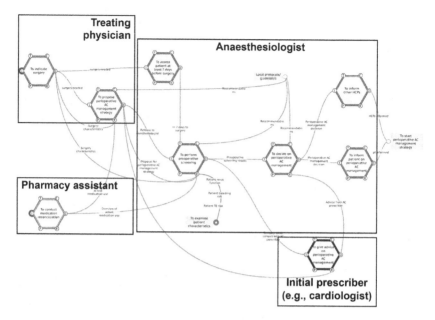

FIGURE 8.1 FRAM model of preoperative anticoagulation management as stipulated by guidelines (i.e., Work-as-Imagined)

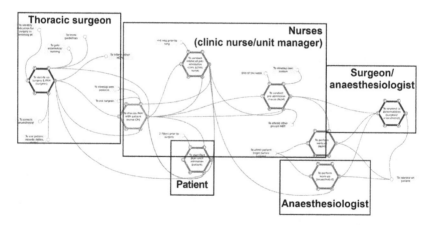

FIGURE 8.2 Work-as-Done FRAM model of preoperative anticoagulation management in the Australian hospital

STAKEHOLDER MEETINGS AND IMPROVEMENT INITIATIVES

Finally, the models are presented to involved staff for validation and discussion. Differences between the process as-imagined and the Work-as-Done can be discussed. In dialogue, involved stakeholders explore to what extent good practices in the process can be strengthened and which improvement initiatives – feasible and suitable in the eyes of those actually carrying out the work – can be thought of to make everyday success more likely.

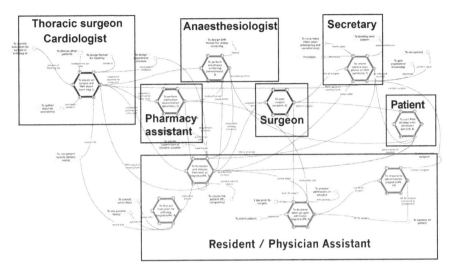

FIGURE 8.3 Work-as-Done FRAM model of preoperative anticoagulation management in the Dutch hospital

USING FRAM TO REVEAL MUDDLING THROUGH-LIKE BEHAVIOUR

In our view, one of the main reasons for FRAM being a powerful tool is that it enables to identify muddling through-like behaviours of professionals. Exactly this muddling reflects adaptive, resilient behaviours and flexibility, which often ensures that a process goes right despite challenging and ever-changing circumstances. To illustrate, we provide some examples of muddling behaviours we encountered in our FRAM analyses.

MUDDLING THROUGH WITH WORKAROUNDS

In daily practice, professionals tend to adapt to unexpected situations all the time, hereby coming up with creative solutions to ensure safe care. For example, one of the junior clinical doctors in our study on preoperative anticoagulation management (Damen et al., 2018) explained that he would always provide patients with a prescription for bridging therapy covering a much longer period of time than initially required. He did so because, in his experience, planned surgeries are often postponed, resulting in patients needing to get a new prescription to cover the additional waiting time. Another example in the same study included the fact that the surgeon and cardiologist chose to not fill in the 'anticoagulation field' in the electronic form specifically designed for their meeting, unless the patient case would require something out of the ordinary. They were unaware of the fact that this behaviour conditioned those using the form later on in the process, to not look at this specific field because it was never filled in anyway. In our experience, professionals very easily reveal these workarounds in a FRAM interview. This may be related to the fact that a FRAM analysis is aimed at assessing everyday practice, rather than a specific case with a negative outcome, which comes with a lot of negative emotions for the interviewee, such as shame and self-blame. In addition, workarounds often become 'common practice' for interviewees as they carry them out everyday, so they might no longer be aware of the fact that these behaviours differ from what was originally imagined.

MUDDLING THROUGH USING PERSONAL AIDS

Almost every analysis of Work-as-Done reveals control mechanisms to ensure successful behaviour, such as critical review of colleagues' decisions and documents or individual systems to enhance efficiency and thoroughness. In interviews, it turned out that professionals who come up with these methods often do so on their own initiative, hence the term 'naturally developed'. For example, in our FRAM analyses we often encountered self-developed checklists, protocols, or notebooks to get a grip on complex processes. Because these methods are often considered 'personal aids', they are not likely to be shared with other (new) staff members. Therefore, these otherwise useful aids can pose problems when key persons are absent or replaced and colleagues are unfamiliar with these personal methods. To illustrate, the secretary we interviewed in our study on anticoagulation management mentioned that she did not plan on handing her self-developed checklist for planned surgeries over to her successor because she considered it 'an old woman's habit' (Damen et al., 2018).

MUDDLING THROUGH WITH UNCLEAR OR UNPRACTICAL ROLES

Guidelines represented in Work-as-Imagined models often suggest specific disciplines to play a central role in a process, while in the Work-as-Done other key figures often carry out these tasks. This exchange of roles may have practical purposes, such as a person who needs to carry out a certain process step will get involved in the preparation phase. Some illustrative examples from our FRAM analysis on preoperative anticoagulation management:

- According to the guidelines and hence our Work-as-Imagined, physicians – and especially anaesthetists – are supposed to play a central role in anticoagulation management around surgery. In practice, however, this appeared to be the responsibility of surgical staff rather than anaesthesia staff, with key roles assigned to (specialised) nurses, registrars and/or physician assistants, who were not mentioned in any guideline but in fact coordinating most of the process;
- Interviewed surgeons felt responsible for formulating and documenting the preoperative anticoagulation strategy for each patient, but other staff reported that this was often omitted in practice, in which case they made the decision instead;

- In contrast to the guidelines, the Dutch hospital did not communicate with out-of-hospital anticoagulation services, usually responsible for outpatient anticoagulation management in the Netherlands. Instead, the department temporarily took over this responsibility until postoperative discharge, in an attempt to prevent confusion for the patient about who was in charge of anticoagulation therapy management.

These examples illustrate how studying Work-as-Done does not only help to identify potential differences between local practices and guidelines, but also the pragmatic, practical reasons behind it.

USABILITY OF FRAM

FRAM appeared to be a promising tool that can be readily applied to study a (complex) health care process, such as medication management, and identify functions that are important for success. We estimate the workload of a FRAM analyses to be about 47 hours per analysis, which is comparable to the workload associated with traditional methods, such as a root-cause analysis (RCA) (Taitz, et al., 2010). Further, clinicians seem to easily understand the relevance, background, and design of FRAM. Reflection meetings with staff are considered insightful and raise awareness of interdependencies between activities of colleagues. Staff also uses the models to discuss opportunities for improvement. This way, FRAM may be used to reconcile and improve the synergy between the world of guidelines and systems design (Work-as-Imagined) and the world of everyday clinical practice (Work-as-Done). Moreover, FRAM models can trigger a discussion on how the fact that each team member 'muddles through with purpose' ensures that the system performs resiliently and successfully.

SUGGESTED FRAMEWORK FOR FRAM MODEL INTERPRETATION

As aforementioned, FRAM models are easily understood by involved professionals, who often recognise the models' visual representation of their daily work. However, after model validation in a staff meeting, the in-depth analysis of the model remains a difficult process, for which the FRAM handbooks provide only little guidance. Based on our experience, we propose a few steps to aid the translation of FRAM models to plans for practical improvements.

Because of the fact that the same 'themes' and muddling behaviours emerged in all FRAM analyses that we have conducted so far, we suggest a framework with four perspectives to interpret and structure FRAM findings:

(1) *Task division and role clarity*
   This theme explores professionals' perceptions of who is responsible for what step (function) in the process, and whether this is clear to and the same for everyone involved. For example, if a cardiologist and cardiothoracic surgeon together decide that a shared patient requires surgery, who is

responsible to make sure that the list of medications in the patient's file is accurate and up to date?

(2) *Multidisciplinary collaboration*

How do involved professionals collaborate in the process? Do they for example have multidisciplinary meetings, or does consultation arise spontaneously?

(3) *Efficiency*

How efficient is the process? Our FRAM analyses showed various work-arounds that ensured safe care but could hamper process efficiency. For example, involved professionals in our anticoagulation study were carrying out the same step in the process at the same time, without knowing this from each other (Damen et al., 2018). Another example includes process features specially designed to optimise the process that were not being used by people on the sharp end.

(4) *Guidance and support*

Are there any protocols/procedures/work agreements used to guide the process? Does everyone use these in the same way (or not at all)? How is supervision of juniors arranged?

In stakeholder meetings, the FRAM model can be presented and discussed using these four perspectives. In our experience so far, they are recognisable for professionals and help them to appreciate what visualisation of their daily work can offer. In addition, the framework guides the development of improvement initiatives. Future studies are needed to further investigate this suggested framework and its effects on longer-term outcomes.

STRENGTHS OF FRAM

Based on our experiences with using FRAM in health care, we have identified the following strengths of the method:

- Insight into Work-as-Done stimulates an 'open' discussion on process design and improvement initiatives. In our view, this leads to a completely different discussion on quality and safety matters, with a more positive and appreciative spirit as well as a more process-based rather than case-based focus, compared to when traditional approaches are used, which mostly focus on cases with negative outcomes;
- The FRAM model is easy to understand by health care professionals. In contrast to reports of a specific case analysis, the FRAM model can be used over again to evaluate a work process, for example, when a new incident occurs or to guide an initiative to make changes to the process;
- Regarding the time investment of a FRAM analysis, there is a bit of a learning curve. But it is our impression that the time it takes to do a FRAM analysis decreases with experience, which makes the method comparable – or even more efficient – than the more traditional quality and safety instruments.

CHALLENGES OF FRAM

As with all methods, besides strengths, FRAM also has some challenges. These are mostly related to the fact that the method is still rather novel, and more scientific research about it is warranted. There is a paucity of comparative research that demonstrates the superiority of this method to more traditional methods. Also, it is important to stress that users are to gain thorough understanding of the underlying theory, especially because FRAM is a 'method without a model'. This introduces the risk that people design a FRAM model and then seek for 'root-causes' of unintended situations and errors, asking 'how this may go wrong', instead of applying the Safety-II approach of seeking ways to make everyday success more likely. In addition, since the method does not provide a clear 'root-cause', it may be difficult for some people to accept that the final product (the FRAM model) does not provide all the answers. Nonetheless, the FRAM model serves as a starting point for reflection and discussion, and this starting point is closer to the reality of everyday practice than looking at a specific situation through the lens of 'Work-as-Imagined'.

CONCLUSION AND FUTURE PERSPECTIVES

To conclude, FRAM provides a useful Safety-II tool to visualise a process in everyday clinical practice that is well received and understood by health care professionals. The method allows identification of functions that are important in daily work and provides the base for feasible and practical improvement initiatives, suitable to the actual situation at the workplace. We proposed a framework to structure and assess the findings of FRAM analyses. More research is warranted to further investigate the usability of FRAM, and its efficacy and efficiency on quality and safety issues.

REFERENCES

Clay-Williams, R., Hounsgaard, J., Hollnagel, E. (2015). Where the rubber meets the road: Using FRAM to align Work-as-Imagined with Work-as-Done when implementing clinical guidelines. *Implementation Science*, 10, 125.

Damen, N. L., de Vos, M. S., Moesker, M.J., Braithwaite, J., de Lind van Wijngaarden, R. A. F., Kaplan, J., … Clay-Williams, R. (2018). Preoperative anticoagulation management in everyday clinical practice: An international comparative analysis of Work-as-Done using the Functional Resonance Analysis Method. *Journal of Patient Safety*. [Epublication ahead of print]. 10.1097/PTS.0000000000000515.

Hollnagel, E., Hounsgaard, J., & Colligan, L. (2014). *FRAM – the Functional Resonance Analysis Method – A Handbook for the Practical Use of the Method*. Region of Southern Denmark: Centre for Quality. Retrieved 22 June 2020, from https://functionalresonance.com/onewebmedia/FRAM_handbook_web-2.pdf.

Hounsgaard, J. (2016). *Patient Safety in Everyday Work. Learning From What Goes Right*. (Master's Thesis, University of Southern Denmark, Odense, Denmark). Retrieved 22 June 2020, from http://functionalresonance.com/onewebmedia/Hounsgaard%20(2016).pdf.

O'Hara, J. K., Baxter, R., & Hardicre, N. (2020). 'Handing over to the patient': A FRAM analysis of transitional care combining multiple stakeholder perspectives. *Applied Ergonomics*, 85, 103060.

Raben, D. C., Viskum, B., Mikkelsen, K. L., Hounsgaard, J., Bogh, S. B., & Hollnagel, E. (2018). Application of a non-linear model to understand healthcare processes: Using the functional resonance analysis method on a case study of the early detection of sepsis. *Reliability Engineering and System Safety*, 177, 1–11.

Taitz, J., Genn, K., Brooks, V.,Ross, D., Ryan, K., Shumack, B., ... NS RCA Review Committee. (2010). System-wide learning from root cause analysis: A report from the New South Wales Root Cause Analysis Review Committee. *Quality and Safety in Health Care*, 19, e63.

9 Modelling a Typical Patient Journey Through the Geriatric Evaluation and Management Ward to Better Understand Discharge Planning Processes

Elizabeth Buikstra, Robyn Clay-Williams and Edward Strivens

CONTENTS

INTRODUCTION

With the increasing complexity associated with the health care system, the ability for health care workers to adjust to match conditions will become increasingly important for sustaining satisfactory performance. The challenge for achieving improvements in safety is to understand how performance usually goes right despite the ambiguities, uncertainties and goal conflicts that permeate the complex health care environment (Hollnagel, Wears, & Braithwaite, 2015).

An analysis method developed by Erik Hollnagel (2012) called the *Functional Resonance Analysis Method* provides a way to describe outcomes using the idea of resonance arising from the variability of everyday performance. This functional resonance is the detectable signal that emerges from the unintended interaction of the normal variabilities of many signals (Hollnagel, 2012). For example, when people complete a task, their performance varies in little ways – perhaps in the time to complete the task or in the steps that are taken. From the viewpoint of an individual, these little variations are not particularly noticeable, and rarely affect the outcome. However, when many people are involved in completing a task, especially when they are dependent on each other for information or other inputs to complete their component of the task, the small individual variations can interact producing exaggerated outcomes or 'resonances'. These resonances can sometimes be helpful, but other times can interfere with smooth performance of the task, resulting in unwanted effects ranging from minor delays or annoyances to serious adverse events.

These small individual variations or incremental adjustments are akin to Charles Lindblom's trial and error process of 'muddling through' (Lindblom, 1959). Lindblom described the method as *successive limited comparisons* or the *branch method* which has the individual 'continually building out from the current situation, step-by-step and by small degrees' (Lindblom, 1959, p. 81). It involves the 'gradual tweaking of experience to balance between the stability of things that have worked in the past and the need to adapt to changing circumstances' (Flach, 2012, p. 195). Lindblom outlined this process as a particular type of decision-making method that was superior when compared to any other decision-making method available for complex problems in many circumstances (Lindblom, 1959).

In hospitals, discharge planning for the older person is complex, with multiple task interactions and multiple opportunities for things to go right and to go wrong (Bauer, Fitzgerald, Haesler, & Manfrin, 2009). Identifying the variability inherent in everyday practice during discharge processes for the older person will assist us in understanding how clinicians 'muddle through' to meet organisational goals and patient needs. By ascertaining what processes are working well, we can also identify potential problem areas in the system's functioning. Our study aimed to describe the discharge planning processes of a typical admission to a Geriatric Evaluation and Management (GEMS) Ward at a regional hospital in Australia. We sought to identify those key features or activities that work well and could mitigate the risk of an adverse event within a typical admission.

METHOD

FUNCTIONAL RESONANCE ANALYSIS METHOD (FRAM)

The purpose of this analysis approach is to provide a concise and methodical representation of 'normal' work as it usually takes place (Work-as-Done). The FRAM is a systematic approach that represents how a dynamic set of actions typically occur (Hollnagel, Hounsgaard, & Colligan, 2014). The selected actions are described in terms of the functions that are necessary to carry out the activity, the potential couplings between the functions, and the typical variability of the functions (Hollnagel et al., 2014). Each function in the model is illustrated by a hexagon surrounded by six aspects (Figure 9.1).

A FRAM analysis is prepared in five steps. These are (0) Determine the purpose and scope of the analysis, (1) Identify and describe the functions, (2) Describe potential and actual performance variability, (3) Aggregation of performance variability, and (4) Propose ways to control variability (Hollnagel, 2012).

Step 0 The Purpose and Scope of the Analysis

The initial step 0 determines the scope and purpose of the analysis and helps to define what work needs to be done. For this study, the FRAM sought to model everyday work to inform understanding of how the adjustments affect the discharge processes for patients on the GEMS ward.

Step 1 Describe Potential and Actual Performance Variability

For this step, the required functions in the work situation are identified and data for describing the functions are collected through semi-structured interviews from staff performing the actual work. Initially, we identified the functions through a *document review and a focus group*. The document review provided information on the formal processes for discharge planning (Work-as-Imagined). Two initial Work-as-Imagined FRAM models were developed using a local Discharge Planning and Estimated Date of Discharge Procedure. The Work-as-Imagined models were presented to a focus

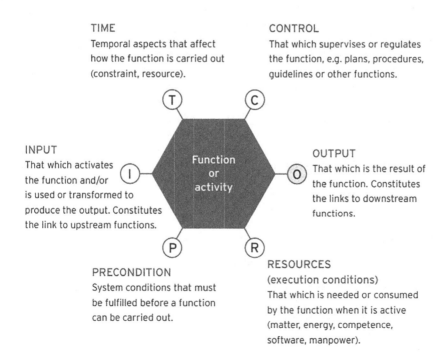

FIGURE 9.1   The six aspects of a function (Hollnagel et al., 2014)

group, which highlighted the limitations and inadequacy of the procedures in describing work as it is usually done on the ward. The group came to a consensus on the functions used for the Work-as-Done discharge planning model. These are described in the Results Section. We then described the *functions* through semi-structured interviews with staff working on the GEMS ward. To describe Work-as-Done in health care, the main source of data should come from experienced people doing the actual work. In this study, the sample of participants were 15 experienced staff working on the ward including three medical officers, three nurses, five allied health practitioners, and two administration officers (AOs). The questions for the interviews focussed on daily activities, routines, habits and practices, and their characteristic variabilities within the ward. The FRAM model was then built and modified based on the data gathered from the interviews and was considered complete when there were no 'loose' aspects. This model was presented to a second focus group who then validated the FRAM model; the final version is described in detail in the Results Section.

Step 2 Describe Potential and Actual Performance Variability

For this step, instantiations of the FRAM model are prepared, showing how the functions are coupled under given conditions. Hollnagel (2009) argues that the trade-off between efficiency and thoroughness can result in performance variability of functions. This variability can propagate through the system, whereby sometimes it is dampened and sometimes becomes abnormally large, creating resonance. Using the FRAM model to predict functional resonance by illustrating how the functions can couple under certain conditions is called an instantiation. Many instantiations are possible in a given model. Each instantiation models couplings between upstream and downstream functions at a given time and for given conditions. Instantiations of the GEMS discharge model are described in detail in the Results Section.

Step 3 Aggregation of Performance Variability and Step 4 Propose Ways to Control Variability

In these steps, the possible outcomes for a given instantiation are assessed to understand how variability can either increase (functional resonance) or decrease (dampened). Recommendations for actions, effective control strategies or monitoring are then developed. The focus of this chapter is the key aspects or functions within the GEMS discharge model that help to dampen functional resonance which could lead to uncontrolled performance variability and ultimately to unwanted outcomes.

RESULTS

The first focus group agreed on four functions to describe Work-as-Done on the GEMS ward: (1) to identify the discharge plan, (2) to organise supports that the patient requires, (3) to ready the patient for discharge and (4) to discharge the patient from the ward. The process for developing the model has been described in detail elsewhere (Buikstra, Strivens, & Clay-Williams, 2020). The model, illustrated as Figure 9.2, is a *typical* admission to the ward and begins with the function 'to refer the patient' and shows how the functions in the discharge planning process depend on each other and interrelate. The functions have been clustered by the colours of

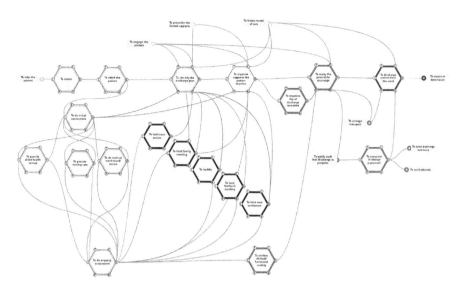

FIGURE 9.2   A FRAM model of the 'typical' admission and discharge planning processes on the GEMS ward

white, black or shades of grey to enhance the interpretation of the model. The functions that are coloured light grey represent those typical processes that flow into and contribute to the preparation of the discharge plan. These include the referral, intake, admission, assessment and care of the patient. The black functions represent the major staffing resources that are usually required for both the discharge plan and organising any supports that the patient requires for discharge. These include family meetings, case review, feedback meetings, huddles and case conferences. The functions with an outline only (white) represent the processes involved in and that generally influence the organisation of supports the patient requires. These include the model of care, patient engagement and the prescription of the formal supports that the patient will require for discharge. These can include Transition Care Programme (TCP) packages, Aged Care packages (in Australia these are called My Aged Care packages), Aged Care Assessment Team evaluations and residential care placements. The medium grey functions represent those functions primarily related to readying the patient for discharge, such as organising the day of discharge resources, completing discharge paperwork and confirming the patient's clinical and functional stability. The functions coloured a darker shade of grey relate to the patient discharging from the ward. For example, one function relates to the patient requiring transport be arranged prior to leaving the ward.

DESCRIBING THE CLUSTERS

As discharge planning is a complex process with many functions depending on each other and interrelating, it seemed prudent to break the GEMS discharge model into sections to improve its interpretability and provide more detail within the model. The following sections provide comprehensive descriptions, including the aspect labels, of the clusters in Figure 9.2. Some of the figures include additional functions that are not from the same cluster. This allows the reader to view the dependencies and inter-relationships among the relevant functions.

CLUSTER 1: TO PREPARE THE PRELIMINARY DISCHARGE PLAN

This process involves the typical activities involved in the development of the pre-liminary discharge plan. The process is described below and in Figure 9.3.

To Refer the Patient
A referral can be received through several methods, including electronically, fax, phone calls, or through paper in the mail. The intake nurse will screen the patient for suitability prior to the referral being given to the Intake Team to assess.

To Intake
The Intake Team hold multidisciplinary meetings Monday to Friday at 11.30 am. Acceptance can occur by medical/nursing or medical/allied health staff. As long as a medical officer is involved, the patient can be determined as suitable and accepted to the ward. The intake review and initial discharge plan is noted in an Intake Workbook.

To Admit the Patient
If the patient is suitable, they will be admitted the same day or as soon as practicable. The nurse involved in the intake assessment will document in the electronic medical

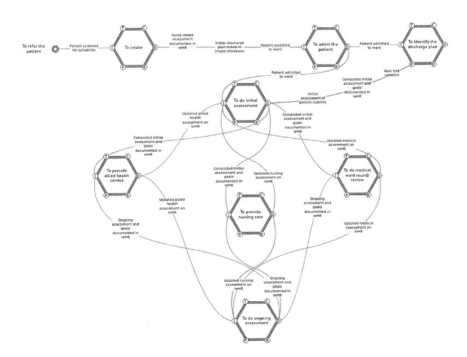

FIGURE 9.3 FRAM model of typical activities involved the development of the preliminary discharge plan

record. The output for the admission is the patient arriving on the ward, in readiness for a full assessment and care by all health professions.

To Do Initial Assessment

The initial assessment is typically a comprehensive assessment of the patient by all professions. It includes the comprehensive care plan, and preliminary work on supports, estimated date of discharge, and discharge destination. The medical officer will assess for medical stability before some specified discharge planning can start, for example, some age care assessments cannot be commenced while a patient is unwell. The allied health assessment includes the completion of a goal tree. The output for the initial assessment by all health professions is a completed initial assessment with goals documented in the electronic medical record, a patient board that has a goal tree updated, as well as the patient's stability to complete rehabilitation. This is all information used in the compilation of the initial discharge plan.

To Provide Allied Health Service/To Provide Nursing Care/To Do Medical Ward Round/Review

Each health profession will provide care and treatment for the patient and document in the electronic medical record. This information will contribute to the preparation of the discharge plan.

To Do Ongoing Assessment

Throughout the patient's admission, each health professional will review their assessment and update the discharge plan based on any changes to the patient's circumstances or condition.

To Identify the Discharge Plan

The discharge plan is formulated once the patient has been admitted to the ward. Staff will engage with the patient, complete an initial assessment of the patient's stability to undertake a rehabilitation programme. All health professions will complete an initial assessment of the patient's goals and document these in the electronic medical record and on a goal tree located in the patient's room. Formal supports, such as referral for Aged Care packages will also be discussed and considered. The initial assessments and comprehensive care plans will be discussed at the weekly case conference. Several outputs occur as a result of the case conference. After the case conference, the patient or their carer will confirm their agreement with the preliminary discharge plan. The output for this function is the estimated discharge date and preliminary discharge plan documented electronically. The information from this function will be utilised by staff when they are organising any supports that the patient may require for discharge.

CLUSTER 2: THE RESOURCES REQUIRED FOR THE DISCHARGE PLAN AND PATIENT SUPPORTS POST-DISCHARGE

This next cluster of functions involves the major staffing resources that are usually required for both the discharge plan and organising any supports that the patient requires for discharge. Each of these resources provides information for the formulation of the discharge plan and required supports. These are illustrated in Figure 9.4.

To Hold Case Review

This is an ad hoc meeting required for individual patients with complex needs. Sensitive issues that have been uncovered during assessments will be discussed. It is particularly important to discuss any legal issues that have been revealed. This information is for the treating team only and will not be discussed during the case conference.

To Hold Family Meeting

This meeting is organised by the social worker and is a crucial component of the discharge plan. There will be a pre-meeting before the family meeting to discuss the plan for the meeting. Engagement with the patient/family/carer/guardian is crucial for the rehabilitation process and identified residential placement.

To Huddle

This meeting is held on a Monday and Wednesday, and includes medical, nursing and allied health staff. This group can make the decision that the patient is ready for early discharge. At the meeting, the patient board is updated with planned family meetings, discharge destination, estimated date of discharge (EDD), and any referrals to the TCP. The electronic management system called Patient Flow Manager (PFM) is

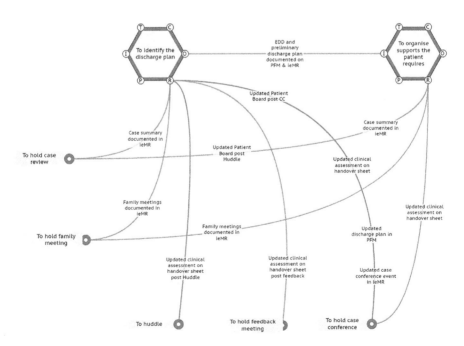

FIGURE 9.4 FRAM model of the resources required for the discharge plan and the supports required for discharge

updated but is not generally used after the huddle but will be printed out the next morning for handover.

To Hold Case Conference

The meeting is held to review the patient's assessment, confirm patient's capacity to consent and their medical stability, confirm supports and review timeframe for EDD and discharge destination. It is held every Thursday between 12.30 and 4.30 pm. The very first case conference for the patient will enable the formulation of a very broad description of the discharge plan with the outcomes documented in various locations, including a handover sheet, patient board, electronic system (PMF), and in the electronic medical record (i.e., EMR).

To Hold Feedback Meeting

This meeting includes nursing and allied health staff and is held on a Tuesday and Friday. The participants will discuss patients from overnight and identify if anything has affected the discharge planning. No major decisions will occur at these meetings. However, the decision to 'stop' a discharge will occur if the acuity of a patient has changed. For example, the patient has had a fall or a stroke overnight.

Cluster 3: Major Influences on the Discharge Plan and the Supports for the Patient Post Discharge

These functions represent the processes that influence the precision and timeliness of the discharge plan and organising any patient supports required for discharge. These include the process of engaging with the patient, the model of care, and the prescription of the formal supports that the patient will require for discharge. Figure 9.5 illustrates this cluster.

To Engage the Patient

Engaging the patient is one of the controlling functions and the most important factor for enabling a timely discharge for the patient. Stakeholders include the patient/

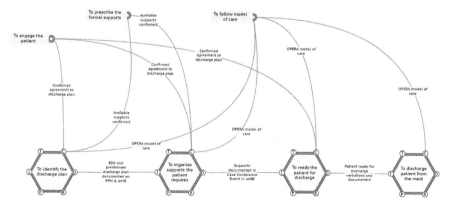

FIGURE 9.5 FRAM model of the major influences on the discharge plan, patient post-discharge supports, and discharging the patient

family/carer/guardian and their buy-in or engagement with the rehabilitation process and identified placement. Without buy-in from these stakeholders the information required for discharge can be inaccurate, or the process can be slowed or even stalled.

To Prescribe the Formal Supports

Prescribing the formal supports for the patient is a complex process and is identified as part of the assessment process. It includes assessing the patient's eligibility and/or suitability for external supports such as the TCP and My Aged Care packages. It may involve aged care assessments and assessment for residential care placement. The patient's stay in hospital is dependent on the process for assessing and organising formal external supports.

To Follow the Model of Care

Another control for discharge planning is that the team will *follow a model of care* that is individualised and person-centric. The entire team is cognisant that they are all striving towards discharge. The model of care influences the entire patient journey, from admission to discharge. There were also comments that an increasing number of older people are presenting acutely unwell with more cognitive impairment, frailer and with less supports. This has placed more pressure on the staff and the model of care.

CLUSTER 4: READYING THE PATIENT FOR DISCHARGE

These are the functions that are crucial to getting the patient ready for discharge. They are illustrated in Figure 9.6.

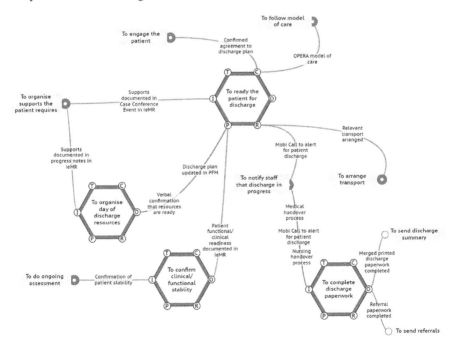

FIGURE 9.6 FRAM model of the key functions to readying the patient for discharge

To Organise Day of Discharge Resources

This is a final check that the resources and supports are ready for the patient to safely discharge home. They include medications (usually webster packs that require 24 hours' notice), prescriptions, placements, out-of-hospital or community supports/referrals have been accepted and equipment. The readiness of supports will have been documented in the medical record. The output for this function is the verbal confirmation that resources are ready, and the discharge plan has been updated in the electronic systems.

To Confirm Clinical/Functional Stability

This is the assessment of the patient's medical stability as well as confirm their ability to manage post-discharge. In addition to medical clearance, the confirmation also requires allied health and nursing clearance. The nursing team leader will review the patient's stability before confirming with the hospital bed managers that the patient is ready to go.

To Notify Staff that Discharge is in Progress

The AO will identify which patients are leaving from the handover sheet, as well as crosscheck with the clinicians who have attended handover. A Mobi Call (alert via sms) is sent to allied health staff alerting them to the patient being discharged and that discharge documentation is required to be finalised by a certain time. The AO will then check the discharge summary documentation about one hour before discharge to see that it is actioned.

To Complete Discharge Paperwork

Discharge paperwork includes discharge summaries (profession specific and inter-disciplinary), ADL (Activities of Daily Living) score sheet, Administration/Discharge Book, Medication Action Plan and Discharge Checklist. This also includes sending referrals to outpatient departments, scheduled care unit, community hospital interface programme, and the community continence nurse. About an hour before discharge, the AO will check that the allied health discharge summary has been completed. If there is any missing information, the AO will contact the relevant staff member to organise completion. Medical staff complete the referral forms and send directly to the relevant parties. Nursing discharge paperwork, for example, nursing transfer summary and wound care plans, are completed and scanned to the relevant service.

To Arrange Transport

This activity includes any patient transport (Transit Lounge, ambulance or flights). Nursing homes will not generally take patients after lunch. If there is a delay with the ambulance, then this might delay the transfer and the nursing home may not keep a place for the patient (e.g., respite bed). The family are encouraged to collect the patient, otherwise the staff may organise a taxi.

To Ready the Patient for Discharge

There are several functions that couple with this function to ensure that the patient is ready to leave hospital. Throughout the admission, relevant staff will have organised suitable supports for discharge and documented these in the electronic medical record, and these include the supports and resources that are required on the day. On the morning of discharge, the overnight nursing team leader will hand over to the morning nursing team leader that a patient is ready for discharge. The nursing team leader will also assess the patient's ability to manage after discharge. If there are problems, the nursing team leader will find a doctor as soon as they come on duty and the medical team will make the call to stop discharge. For allied health, this relates to any assessments that are required for discharge placement. Engagement with relevant stakeholders (patient/family/carer/guardian) is crucial to ensuring the patient discharges in a safe and timely way.

CLUSTER 5: DISCHARGING THE PATIENT FROM THE WARD

The final part of the discharge process is supporting the patient to leave the hospital. This is represented in Figure 9.7.

To Discharge the Patient from the Ward

The patient is ready to be discharged from the ward when discharge resources and documentation are ready, and the patient's transport has been arranged. With all staff focussed on a safe and timely discharge, the model of care is a major influencing factor in this activity. The patient will leave the ward with a nursing transfer summary. This summary will also be sent electronically, along with the discharge paperwork from the other health professionals to the relevant receiving service (TCP, residential care, outlying facility).

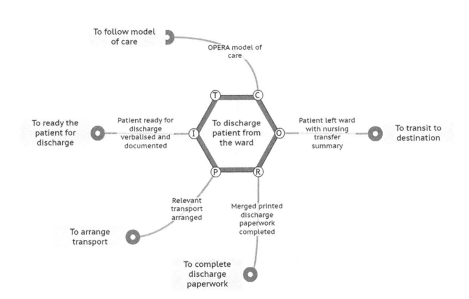

FIGURE 9.7   FRAM model of the functions involved in discharging the patient from the ward

To Transit to Destination

The patient can be picked up by their family, a staff member from the TCP, or transported to the hospital Transit Lounge (interim wait for final discharge from the hospital). The patient can be discharged to home/family, residential care, or an outlying facility.

RISK OF FUNCTIONAL RESONANCE AND DAMPENING THE PERFORMANCE VARIABILITY

Four key instantiations were identified when modelling a typical admission to the GEMS ward. These are described in relation to the uncontrolled performance variability that might lead to unwanted outcomes, and the positive features or activities that have contributed to dampening this variability.

Missed Referrals

Referrals can be made via several methods. The clinical staff are mindful of the multiple referral entry points and check regularly. While it was identified during the interviews that this could be streamlined to one or two entry points, the staff wanted to ensure that the patient would not be excluded based on the referral method. All referrals are screened by the intake nurse and the intake team. This comprehensive process and part of the GEMS discharge planning model of care ensures that suitable patients are accepted to the ward. The risk of functional resonance relates to a delay in the patient's admission to the ward if their referral is initially missed (performance variability). This has the potential for extending the length of stay if the patient's condition has further deteriorated prior to admission. Positive relationships and good communication with staff in the hospital and community dampen the variability associated with a missed referral, that is, referrers are encouraged to contact clinical staff to discuss a referral. This is an essential feature developed as part of the model of care for the ward.

Missing Information from Intake

After the patient review was completed by the Intake Team, the initial discharge plan was noted in the Intake Workbook. This information was documented in a separate spreadsheet of which only the Intake Team have access. Interview participants identified that the intake information was crucial for clinical staff in their assessment of the patient and development of a comprehensive care and discharge plan. The risk of functional resonance arises when plans are developed based on the information in the electronic medical record and the patient's own desires which could be inconsistent with the Intake Team's goals for admission (performance variability). This could lead to an inaccurate estimated date of discharge and the risk of extending the patient's length of stay. This performance variability has been recognised and mitigated by the Intake Medical Officer writing a summary of the intake assessment and initial discharge plan into the electronic medical record post-intake.

Delayed Assessments to Enable Formulation of the Discharge Plan

Allied health staff indicated that their assessments were not always completed in time for the weekly case conference. This is the main forum in which the discharge plan is developed. The risk of functional resonance arises as the planning process may not have considered crucial information from a specific allied health professional's assessment (performance variability). Length of stay in hospital could be extended as a result. However, as medical and nursing assessments will be available, a broad formulation of the discharge plan can be developed and modified in the weeks that follow. To dampen the performance variability, the development of the discharge plan during the case conference is usually completed in collaboration with the allied health staff who can provide input based on their experience with similar conditions. This collaborative approach features in all aspects of the interdisciplinary team model of care.

Delayed Notification of Pending Discharge

Allied health staff receive an electronic notification from the AO to complete their discharge summaries. Nursing and medical staff have traditionally relied on the usual handover processes as a reminder to complete their discharge summaries. The risk of functional resonance arises when paperwork is not completed in a timely manner (performance variability). There can be a delay in discharge summaries being distributed to the patient and relevant health practitioners, which can result in inadequate post-discharge treatment and care. To dampen the performance variability, agreement was reached that all clinical staff receive an electronic notification from the AO, with subsequent follow up from the AO for timely completion.

KEY FEATURES THAT DAMPEN UNCONTROLLED PERFORMANCE VARIABILITY

Three key features were noted to contribute to dampening the variability in the four instantiations.

Model of Care

Throughout the process, the staff emphasised that the GEMS discharge model of care was paramount to the patient being discharged in a safe and timely manner. Participants described the interdisciplinary model of care as individualised and person-centric, with the principal goal of safe discharge for the patient. As staff are all striving toward discharge, this interdisciplinary model of care influences the entire patient journey toward discharge.

Engagement with the Patient

Ward staff work particularly hard and spend the time and effort to engage with the patient, carer, family and/or guardian. Engaging with the patient includes one-on-one health care assessment, review, care, education and therapy, as well as family meetings with the health care team to discuss the discharge plan. Without successful buy-in or engagement, there is a risk that the discharge will fail. The health care team will emphasise the importance of the patient/carer/family and ensuring that they understand the role that they play in a successful discharge in the longer term.

Daily Communication and Sharing of Information

To ensure that all relevant health professionals are kept up to date on the patient's care and discharge status, meetings are held daily. These include huddles on Monday and Wednesday, feedback meetings on Tuesday and Friday, and case conference on Thursday. Nursing and allied health staff are involved in each of these meetings, with medical staff involved in the huddles and case conference. If medical input is required on a Tuesday or Friday, consultation with a medical officer will occur after the meeting.

DISCUSSION

Hospital discharge planning for the older person is complex with many opportunities for the discharge plan to go right and to go wrong, and performance can have unintended consequences, such as an adverse event or patient harm (Bauer et al., 2009). There is inherent variability in everyday practice on the ward and understanding this helps to understand how clinicians typically 'muddle through' to meet the organisation's and patients' needs. We achieved our aim of describing the discharge planning processes of a typical admission to identify key aspects that work well and could mitigate the risk of an adverse event.

The concept of 'muddling through' provides a framework for understanding how the individual when faced with a complex problem, finds a way to drastically simplify it (Lindblom, 1959). In other words, the framework allows for complex problems which cannot be completely analysed to be analysed with skilful incompleteness (Lindblom, 1979). While Lindblom (1959, 1979) refers to policymaking in public administration, his theoretical method of 'muddling through' can be applied to similarly complex issues such as the formulation of a discharge plan for a frail older person within the context of a complicated hospital and health care environment. The application of this method in the discharge planning process includes the progression of successive approximations and decisions toward the desired objective of safe and timely patient discharge with appropriate supports, with the discharge plan itself continuing to be reviewed and modified throughout the admission. This 'incremental adjustment' or *incrementalism*, if completed skilfully, has increasing support from the research community with normative models of decision and choice not able to be realised in this type of complex problem space (Flach, 2012). Flach (2012) describes this type of incrementalism as the skill of balancing between the experience of what has worked in the past and an openness to learn from mistakes and unexpected events that are inevitable in a complex environment. This was evident throughout the interviews and in the development of the FRAM model where staff were able to consistently identify what was working well and reflect on what went wrong in the discharge planning process. The GEMS discharge model was broken down into five clusters to enhance the interpretability of the model and to show how the functions flow into and contribute to the preparation of the discharge plan.

The first cluster involved the typical activities involved in the development of the discharge plan and revealed three opportunities for functional resonance or uncontrolled performance variability that might lead to unwanted outcomes. Missed referrals, missed information from intake, and delayed assessments can contribute to unwanted outcomes for the patient, such as an extended length of stay. An interdisciplinary team model of care that includes positive patient engagement and effective communication provides the platform for staff to use their experience of what has worked in the past and adjust their decisions when confronted with new information and unexpected events. The interdisciplinary team model of care was also evident as a major feature in the other clusters.

The second cluster involved the staffing resources required for the discharge plan and the supports that the patient will require post-discharge. Effectively communicating and sharing information was found to be an important factor in successful discharge planning in this study. This is consistent with previous research (Carroll & Dowling, 2007). Each staffing resource, that is the case review, family meeting, huddle, case conference and feedback meeting, requires timely and precise communication/information. This is generally represented as an output in the FRAM model. For example, outputs for the case conference include an updated case conference event in the electronic medical record, an updated discharge plan in the electronic system (PFM), an updated clinical assessment on the handover sheet and an updated Patient Board in the central write-up area. This is a broad description of a very complex discharge planning communication process and staff manage the process by constantly tweaking their plans based on their experience of what has worked in the past and the need to adapt to new information they receive. They 'muddle' through.

The third cluster described the major influences on the discharge plan including the model of care, patient engagement and the prescription of formal supports. Our model showed that the GEMS model of care, which was interdisciplinary, person-centric, with tailored individualised discharge planning, was a crucial component of a successful discharge plan. The model of care had the effect of regulating or controlling the major activities throughout the discharge planning process and dampening down any uncontrolled performance variability. This is not a rigid model of care because the flexibility shown by staff allowed for them to make incremental adjustments in their behaviour/decisions throughout the patient's admission which reduced the risk of unexpected events. Further exploration of the success in the GEMS interdisciplinary model of care provides scope for further research. Suggested major features to be explored have been identified in a recent metasynthesis and include: (1) unifying the team for a meaningful purpose, (2) identifying and clarifying roles within the team, (3) having a shared vocabulary, (4) collaboration and integration, (5) the barriers and challenges that the interprofessional team experienced, and (6) client-centred care (Montano, 2020).

Another key feature in the third cluster is the process of engagement with the patient, carer, family and/or guardian. Engaging with the patient involves their active participation in one-on-one assessment, review, care, education and therapy. Working with the patient and their family and incrementally adjusting decisions regarding the discharge plan throughout the admission to meet the patient's needs reduces the likelihood of the discharge failing. A failed discharge usually results in the patient staying unnecessarily longer in hospital. Positive patient engagement affects many activities throughout the discharge planning process and can dampen down uncontrolled performance variability to reduce the risk of an extended length of stay. Involving patients and their family caregivers in their health care journey has been consistently highlighted as a feature of successful interventions (Bull & Roberts, 2001; Coleman, Parry, Chalmers, & Min, 2006; Foss & Hofoss, 2011; Laugaland, Aase, & Barach, 2012; Naylor et al., 1999; Naylor et al., 2004). Indeed, patient-centred care is recognised internationally as a dimension of high-quality health care (Australian Commission on Safety and Quality in Health Care, 2011).

The fourth and fifth clusters related to readying the patient for discharge and supporting them to leave hospital. Review of these clusters revealed another opportunity for functional resonance with the risk of unwanted outcomes. Delayed notification of pending discharge can result in delay in distribution of discharge summaries and the possibility of inadequate post-discharge treatment and care. The opportunity for functional resonance was clearly illustrated using the FRAM model and staff were able to agree on a timely practical solution.

PRACTICAL IMPLICATIONS

The FRAM method and model have highlighted the day-to-day issues that health care staff are confronted with in an environment that is ever-changing. The model illustrated that there were key features of the discharge model, consisting of objectives that needed to be embraced and enhanced, and other aspects that highlighted the performance variability that needed quality improvement. The need to trade-off thoroughness for efficiency drive staff to adopt a muddling through process, whereby objectives are agreed, but the actual process varies to meet patient needs and the demands of the work. The FRAM allowed us to identify the major features of the discharge model of care that help staff to muddle through each and every workday, showing how options are combined and choices made, and indicating where incremental adjustments will have the greatest effect on outcome.

RESEARCH IMPLICATIONS

The current study illustrates how FRAM can be utilised as a research tool in the health care system for better understanding 'Work-as-Done' and how clinicians muddle through in their everyday work to achieve hospital objectives. The methodology can be useful for mapping performance variability in the workplace, including who chooses which path to achieve the organisational aims, with a view to identifying what processes could help to mitigate the risk of patient harm. This model also focussed on the discharge processes while the patient was admitted to hospital. The literature would suggest that post-discharge interventions are also crucial and warrant examination (e.g., Laugaland et al., 2012); therefore, future research could include modelling the discharge support processes after the patient leaves hospital. Another area identified for further examination that was highlighted during interviews, but not included as part of the FRAM model, is the discharge medication processes. Future research could also include the FRAM method as an evaluation tool for local quality improvement interventions.

LIMITATIONS

There are some limitations to this study. Some of these have been identified in a previous paper (Buikstra et al., 2020). One limitation is the inability to translate findings to other hospital wards because the FRAM methodology is designed to enable quality improvements to be tailored to that workplace. Also, the method is based on self-report which relies on the accuracy of participants' memories. To reduce the risk of hindsight bias, several different participants across different professions were asked similar questions. The third limitation cited previously related to the lack of patient involvement in the research. It is noted that previously research on the GEMS ward examined the perceptions of patients and caregivers' experiences of care transitions across different locations and levels of care. Our study focussed on 'Work-as-Done' with one group of health professionals in one setting, at one point in time. This limits the transferability of this qualitative research, however, the lessons learnt from examining the discharge processes might provide health professionals who are working with the older person the opportunity to critically reflect on their own processes and ascertain similar learnings that could be adapted.

REFERENCES

Australian Commission on Safety and Quality in Health Care (ACSQHC). (2011). *Patient-centred care: Improving quality and safety through partnerships with patients and consumers*. Sydney, Australia: ACSQHC.

Bauer, M., Fitzgerald, L., Haesler, E., & Manfrin, M. (2009). Hospital discharge planning for frail older people and their family. Are we delivering best practice? A review of the evidence. *Journal of Clinical Nursing*, 18(18), 2539–2546.

Buikstra, E., Strivens, E., & Clay-Williams, R. (2020). Understanding variability in discharge planning processes for the older person. *Safety Science*, 121, 137–146.

Bull, M. J., & Roberts, J. (2001). Components of a proper hospital discharge for elders. *Journal of Advanced Nursing*, 35(4), 571–581.

Carroll, A., & Dowling, M. (2007). Discharge planning: communication, education and patient participation. *British Journal of Nursing*, 16(14), 882–886.

Coleman, E. A., Parry, C., Chalmers, S., & Min, S-J. (2006). The care transitions intervention: results of a randomized controlled trial. *Archives of Internal Medicine*, 166(17), 1822–1828.

Flach, J. M. (2012). Complexity: learning to muddle through. *Cognition, Technology & Work*, 14(3), 187–197.

Foss, C., & Hofoss, D. (2011). Elderly persons' experiences of participation in hospital discharge process.(Report). *Patient Education and Counseling*, 85(1), 68.

Hollnagel, E. (2009). *The ETTO Principle: Efficiency-Thoroughness Trade-Off – Why Things That Go Right Sometimes Go Wrong*. Surrey, England: Ashgate Publishing.

Hollnagel, E. (2012). *FRAM: The Functional Resonance Analysis Method – Modelling Complex Socio-technical Systems*. Farnham, UK: Ashgate Publishing.

Hollnagel, E., Hounsgaard, J., & Colligan, L. (2014). *FRAM: The Functional Resonance Analysis Method – A Handbook for the Practical Use of the Method*. Retrieved 7 September 2020, from http://functionalresonance.com/onewebmedia/FRAM_handbook_web-2.pdf.

Hollnagel, E., Wears, R. L., & Braithwaite, J. (2015). *From Safety-I to Safety-II: A White Paper*. The resilient health care net: published simultaneously by the University of Southern Denmark, University of Florida, USA, and Macquarie University, Australia.

Laugaland, K., Aase, K., & Barach, P. (2012). Interventions to improve patient safety in transitional care - a review of the evidence. *Work*, 41, 2915–2924.

Lindblom, C. E. (1959). The science of "muddling through". *Public Administration Review*, 19(2), 79–88.

Lindblom, C. E. (1979). Still muddling, not yet through. *Public Administration Review*, 39(6), 517–526.

Montano, A.-R. (2020). "All for One" experiences of interprofessional team members caring for older adults: A metasynthesis. *International Journal of Older People Nursing*, 15(1), e12290.

Naylor, M. D., Brooten, D., Campbell, R., Jacobsen, B. S., Mezey, M. D., Pauly, M. V., & Schwartz, J. S. (1999). Comprehensive discharge planning and home follow-up of hospitalized elders: A randomized clinical trial. *Journal of the American Medical Association*, 281(7), 613–620.

Naylor, M. D., Brooten, D. A., Campbell, R. L., Maislin, G., McCauley, K. M., & Schwartz, J. S. (2004). Transitional care of older adults hospitalized with heart failure: A randomized, controlled trial. *Journal of the American Geriatrics Society*, 52(5), 675–684.

10 Muddling Through in the Intensive Care Unit

A FRAM Analysis of Intravenous Infusion Management

Mark A. Sujan

CONTENTS

INTRODUCTION

In previous contributions to this book series on Resilient Health Care (RHC), I explored how health care workers make dynamic trade-offs, for example, when handing over a patient between an ambulance crew and emergency department staff or when referring a patient from the emergency department to a hospital ward (Sujan, Huang, & Biggerstaff, 2019; Sujan, Spurgeon, & Cooke, 2015b). The reason why this focus on making trade-offs is important is that in any health system there are inherent and inevitable tensions and contradictions, which cannot be designed out, but which require resolution within the context of a specific situation, i.e., a dynamic trade-off. The ability to make such trade-offs is, therefore, a mechanism of resilience and an expression of 'muddling through with purpose'.

The need for trade-offs has been articulated in different ways, for example, via a recourse to complexity science suggesting that modern systems are inherently intractable (Braithwaite, Clay-Williams, Nugus, & Plumb, 2013; Hollnagel, 2014), or via highlighting the mismatch between demand and capacity (Anderson, Ross, & Jaye, 2017). Personally, I align with the notion of tensions and inner contradictions, as expressed in the writings of Vygotsky, Luria and Leontiev, who founded the cultural-historic Activity Theory (Vygotsky, 1978). Activity Theory uses the concept of inner contradictions of an activity. Contradictions are misfits or misalignments within an activity or between activities. The mismatch between demand and capacity could be regarded as one specific case of a contradiction, but the concept of contradictions is more far reaching and can include other expressions, such as competing priorities or goal conflicts where an activity involves multiple people. Contradictions manifest themselves externally as disturbances or disruptions, i.e., as the undesired effects that we perceive. These undesired effects cannot simply be eliminated without addressing the underlying contradiction. However, the fundamental point of the application of dialectics within Activity Theory is that contradictions are enabling change and development (Engestrom, 1987). It is the contradictions that lead to innovations, which in turn inevitably create new contradictions. Readers with an inclination for the philosophical will note that this application of dialectics originates with German philosophers Hegel (applied idealistically) and Marx (applied materialistically), but this philosophical discourse is beyond the scope of the chapter.

The above theoretical outline might sound very abstract, but regardless of the theoretical stance one subscribes to, all of these theories suggest that in modern health systems people, and the systems within which they work, need to adapt what they do (Work-as-Done) rather than just follow rigid work procedures and protocols (Work-as-Imagined). Hence the need for studying how health care workers make trade-offs, so that we can support their ability to make these trade-offs successfully more frequently (Sujan, Spurgeon, & Cooke, 2015a).

What I found in my previous book chapters is that people make dynamic trade-offs based on their experience and based on what could be regarded a subjective and intuitive risk assessment of the current situation. I illustrated this with the example of the 'secret second handover', which describes how paramedics resolve the inherent tensions (or contradiction) between staying with the patient under their care at the hospital until they are satisfied that they have communicated to hospital staff all relevant details and the urgency of leaving the hospital quickly in order to meet the needs of other patients in the community. Interviews with paramedics revealed that they resolve this tension through a very subjective feeling of 'being worried' – when they are worried about their patient, they will wait until they are reassured that they have handed over everything about the patient properly. When they are not worried, they are more inclined to trade-off the other way, and potentially even hand over to another ambulance crew while waiting in a queue outside of the hospital.

Trust (Kramer, 1999) and psychological safety (Edmondson, Kramer, & Cook, 2004) are further factors that influence how health care workers make trade-offs. When referring a patient from the emergency department to hospital wards, the clinicians involved need to negotiate jointly a number of trade-offs, such as reducing overcrowding in the emergency department while ensuring that a full diagnosis is available in order to send the patient to the right ward. How this trade-off is resolved clearly depends on the acuity and condition of the patient, but not just. If there is a level of trust and if people feel safe to take interpersonal risks, then these referral conversations are more likely to be responsive to considerations such as perceived business of the emergency department. If, on the other hand, these factors are missing, then the trade-off is more likely to be resolved according to the (static) protocols, i.e., referrals must have a clear diagnosis. This can lead to behaviours referred to as 'selling patients', which can cause frustration and further distrust (Nugus et al., 2017).

My aim in this chapter is to illustrate how the Functional Resonance Analysis Method (FRAM) might be used to study how health care workers make trade-offs and how FRAM can help with exploring the impact of these trade-offs on other activities. The FRAM (Hollnagel, 2012) probably does not require any further introduction as it is an increasingly well-known technique, but in the next section I give a very brief overview of its key principles and how it can be applied to study trade-offs. Then, I describe the case of intravenous medication management in the intensive care unit (ICU), where FRAM was applied to study how infusions are ordered and administered. I conclude the chapter with a reflection on lessons learned.

FRAM

FRAM is one of the most significant and widely used methods developed within the Resilience Engineering paradigm (Patriarca et al., 2020). FRAM moves away from the assumption that accidents are caused by component failures and human errors. Instead, the thinking behind FRAM suggests that failures can result from dysfunctional interactions, where variability spreads in unexpected ways and is reinforced throughout the system. FRAM is increasingly being used as a prospective analysis method for understanding performance variability in everyday work or Work-as-Done. FRAM has seen widespread uptake especially within health care, where the complexity of everyday clinical work lends itself particularly well to the study with FRAM (Kaya, Ovali, & Ozturk, 2019; Pickup et al., 2017; Raben, Bogh, Viskum, Mikkelsen, & Hollnagel, 2018; Schutijser et al., 2019). Considering the diversity of applications and the various extensions and modifications that different authors have proposed, it is hard to speak of 'the' FRAM as if it were a neatly laid out algorithm. Arguably, this flexibility that allows the method to be used in different ways and with different emphasis is a strength of FRAM. Nonetheless, a FRAM analysis typically consists of these core steps: (1) identification of functions, (2) description of performance variability, (3) analysis of couplings and then (4) managing variability.

Performance variability is often an expression of trade-offs, i.e., health care workers encounter tensions in their everyday work, and they resolve these depending on the context by muddling through with purpose. FRAM can be helpful for the study of performance variability with the aim of understanding how the ability to make trade-offs can be strengthened, and representing how the consequences of muddling through might have consequences elsewhere (either in space or time) in the system.

EXAMPLE: INTRAVENOUS MEDICATION ORDERING

The example is taken from a project that studied safety assurance challenges of the use of autonomous infusion pumps (i.e., infusion pumps driven by artificial intelligence) for intravenous (IV) medication administration in intensive care. FRAM was one of the key methods of investigation. FRAM was used for studying Work-as-Done prior to the introduction of the autonomous technology in order to understand how clinicians anticipate, adapt, monitor and learn as part of everyday clinical work, i.e., how they put resilience abilities into practice. The purpose of doing this was to make recommendations that could feed into the design and implementation of the autonomous technology in such a way that its use enhances rather than diminishes resilience abilities.

The project was carried out in an English NHS hospital. The hospital serves a population of 600,000. It has a capacity of 1,131 beds and employs over 8,800 staff. The ICU within the hospital has 16 beds, and is staffed by approximately 35 medical staff, 100 nurses and 80 support staff. The ICU cares for 1,300 patients annually. The project was concerned with IV medication management systems in the ICU. Patients in ICU are, by default, very ill. Patients can be on life support machines, such as ventilators, and they typically require a significant number of drugs. Some of these drugs are given intravenously via an infusion pump. The infusion pump controls the flow of the drug. The traditional setup is that a doctor (or clinician with prescribing privileges) prescribes a drug as part of the patient's treatment plan, and a nurse then needs to prepare the drug syringe, load the infusion pump with the drug syringe, and then program the infusion pump to run at the required infusion rate for a specific duration. This is the baseline scenario used for illustration in this chapter. A more comprehensive description of the analysis is given in Furniss et al. (2020), and I will only refer to a small part to illustrate the approach.

The FRAM analysis identified 35 separate functions grouped into six clusters of functional activity, see Table 10.1.

Following identification and description of the functions, the analysis involved description of variability as manifestation or as the observable expression of underlying resilience abilities. Hence, observed performance variability was characterised in terms of whether and how it serves as a mechanism of anticipation, adaptation, monitoring or learning. This is reflected in the structure of Table 10.2, which looks at the variability around ordering medication. The analysis of performance variability in this way can provide insights into how health care workers muddle through with purpose.

TABLE 10.1
Functional clusters and functions for intravenous medication management

Functional Cluster	Functions
Medication ordering	Give verbal order; Write new order; Make written change to order; Do medicines reconciliation; Supervise medication management process
Infusion preparation	Check prescription; Gather equipment for preparation; Ensure medications are available and stocked; Gather drugs and fluids; Gather equipment for administration; Do drug calculations; Complete labels; Consult BNF and guidance; Prepare infusion
Interacting with patient	Inform patient about infusion details; Get consent for infusion; Do patient checks; Do visitor-supported checks
Infusion administration	Check current infusions; Go to patient; Check and flush access device; Connect lines; Get pump; Program pump; Release roller clamp; Start pump; Administer medication; Monitor infusion; Stop and disconnect infusion; Flush line; Create plan for change to infusion
Double checking	Double check preparation and administration
Monitoring and documentation	Check previous doses; Monitor patient response; Document infusion

For example, an interesting source of variability for ordering medication is whether it is written (as per clinical protocol, i.e., Work-as-Imagined) or verbal, as this can have a large impact on the process downstream. The benefit of introducing this performance variability (i.e., written or verbal) is that it can deal with different kinds of demands, e.g., a verbal order is very good when there is an urgent need for treating the patient, and conversely a written order provides a clear audit trail and details for nurses to act upon. Verbal orders tend to be in the presence of the patient, e.g., during admission or when the doctor is treating the patient like putting a central line in or giving life support. After patient admission or when the treatment is complete the doctor will often sit down and do the paperwork including the prescription. Another way this variability can arise is when the nurse anticipates or responds to what the patient needs before the doctor does, and then prompts the doctor for this who can then review and write up the medication order later.

Note, that in Table 10.2 I include consideration of variability propagation, but in a non-normative way. The output of a function varies in line with the requirements of

TABLE 10.2

Performance variability in medication ordering

Manifestation of Variability: What was Observed?	Tensions and Uncertain Performance Conditions: How Does this Demonstrate Resilience?	Upstream/Downstream Coupling: What are the Consequences of this Performance Variability?
There could be a written prescription or a verbal order for a drug.	There might be an emergency scenario whereby the drug has to be given immediately, or doctors may be too busy to write an order so advise that the administration proceeds without it (*adaptation*).	In all cases a written order should follow a verbal order. This creates an extra function for the nurse and doctor to *monitor* that a written order follows.
The prescription/order could come before or after the administration.	Nurses may perceive a need for fluids or drugs but the doctors might not have written an order yet. For example, a continuous infusion might need to be officially reordered when the current infusion is ending but the doctors might be unavailable, so the nurse continues it in *anticipation* of an order.	Again, this creates an extra function for the nurse to *monitor* that they follow this up with the doctors and an order follows.
The prescription/order could be very specific and comprehensive about rate, dose, etc.; it could also be more general like ordering 'fluids', or incomplete.	What details are missing, how they are perceived and the demands of the context will impact the *adaptive* strategies chosen: If these are perceived as important then the doctor should be challenged. If not perceived as important the nurse will most likely get on with it and add and/or correct details later if necessary. The urgency of the drug, its potency, and the availability of the doctor might also influence how individuals adapt. There is a trade-off between being efficient (getting on with the task) or being thorough (making sure all information is complete and correct).	Challenging the doctor depends on perceived consequences (e.g., how uneasy the nurse feels about the missing information), and the availability of the doctor (e.g., if they are present or the next bed along the cost is low, if they are away from the ward they could be hard to find and might not like being interrupted).

the situation, and this is subsequently reflected in downstream functions, either in terms of which functions are activated or when they are activated, or in additional functions being created, etc. In this way, FRAM can be a useful tool to reason about the consequences of muddling through. For example, if the medication order is verbal, then it becomes necessary for the nurse to monitor (and potentially remind the doctor) that a written medication order is done at a later point in time. This is represented in FRAM through the creation of new functions.

CONCLUSION

In the example described, FRAM turned out to be an excellent tool for representing Work-as-Done, and for analysing performance variability in order to understand how success is created through resilient forms of behaviour or resilience abilities. Muddling through is done with a purpose, and I suggest that this purpose can be analysed by looking at the dynamic trade-offs that health care workers make in order to deal with tensions and contradictions inherent in their work and systems of work.

I conclude this chapter by acknowledging that this is a job only half done. As we gain greater insights into how people make trade-offs and how the consequences of trade-offs might impact other functions in the system (e.g., by using FRAM), we need to turn our attention to how we strengthen health care workers' ability to make trade-offs. The FRAM analysis can be a useful tool for reflection for those involved in delivering and managing the work, and it can provide guidance for the design of tools and technologies. For example, if the process of intravenous infusion administration is going to be automated, then the outputs of the FRAM analysis can suggest ways in which the automation can be designed so that existing sources of resilience do not get disrupted or that resilience abilities are strengthened. There is a lot of scope for further research in this area.

ACKNOWLEDGEMENTS

This work was supported by the Assuring Autonomy International Programme, a partnership between Lloyd's Register Foundation and the University of York. Dominic Furniss, Shakir Laher, Sean White, Ibrahim Habli, David Nelson, Matthew Elliott and Nick Reynolds were part of the project team.

REFERENCES

Anderson, J. E., Ross, A. J., & Jaye, P. (2017). Modelling resilience and reasearching the gap between Work-as-Imagined and Work-as-Done. In J. Braithwaite, R. Wears, & E. Hollnagel (Eds.), *Resilient Health Care, Volume 3: Reconciling Work-as-Imagined with Work-as-Done* (pp. 166–175). Boca Raton, FL: CRC Press.

Braithwaite, J., Clay-Williams, R., Nugus, P., & Plumb, J. (2013). Healthcare as a complex adaptive system. In E. Hollnagel, J. Braithwaite, & R. Wears (Eds.), *Resilient Health Care* (pp. 57–73). Farnham, UK: Ashgate Publishing.

Edmondson, A. C., Kramer, R. M., & Cook, K. S. (2004). Psychological safety, trust, and learning in organizations: A group-level lens. In K. S. Cook & R. M. Kramer (Eds.), *Trust and Distrust in Organizations: Dilemmas and Approaches* (Vol. 12, pp. 239–272). New York, NY: Russel Sage Foundation.

Engestrom, Y. (1987). *Learning by Expanding: An Activity-Theoretical Approach to Developmental Research.* Helsinki, Finland: Orienta-Konsultit.

Furniss, D., Nelson, D., Habli, I., White, S., Elliott, M., Reynolds, N., & Sujan, M. (2020). Using FRAM to explore sources of performance variability in intravenous infusion administration in ICU: A non-normative approach to systems contradictions. *Applied Ergonomics*, 86, 103113.

Hollnagel, E. (2012). *FRAM, the Functional Resonance Analysis Method: Modelling Complex Socio-technical Systems.* Farnham, UK: Ashgate Publishing.

Hollnagel, E. (2014). *Safety-I and Safety-II. The Past and Future of Safety Mangement.* Farnham, UK: Ashgate Publishing.

Kaya, G. K., Ovali, H. F., & Ozturk, F. (2019). Using the functional resonance analysis method on the drug administration process to assess performance variability. *Safety Science*, 118, 835–840.

Kramer, R. M. (1999). Trust and distrust in organizations: Emerging perspectives, enduring questions. *Annual Review of Psychology*, 50(1), 569–598.

Nugus, P., McCarthy, S., Holdgate, A., Braithwaite, J., Schoenmakers, A., & Wagner, C. (2017). Packaging patients and handing them over: Communication context and persuasion in the emergency department. *Annals of Emergency Medicine*, 69(2), 210–217.e2.

Patriarca, R., Di Gravio, G., Woltjer, R., Costantino, F., Praetorius, G., Ferreira, P., & Hollnagel, E. (2020). Framing the FRAM: A literature review on the functional resonance analysis method. *Safety Science*, 129, 104827.

Pickup, L., Atkinson, S., Hollnagel, E., Bowie, P., Gray, S., Rawlinson, S., & Forrester, K. (2017). Blood sampling – Two sides to the story. *Applied Ergonomics*, 59, 234–242.

Raben, D. C., Bogh, S. B., Viskum, B., Mikkelsen, K. L., & Hollnagel, E. (2018). Learn from what goes right: A demonstration of a new systematic method for identification of leading indicators in healthcare. *Reliability Engineering & System Safety*, 169, 187–198.

Schutijser, B. C. F. M., Jongerden, I. P., Klopotowska, J. E., Portegijs, S., de Bruijne, M. C., & Wagner, C. (2019). Double checking injectable medication administration: Does the protocol fit clinical practice? *Safety Science*, 118, 853–860.

Sujan, M., Huang, H., & Biggerstaff, D. (2019). Trust and psychological safety as facilitators of resilient health care. In J. Braithwaite, E. Hollnagel, & G. Hunte (Eds.), *Resilient Health Care, Volume 5: Working Across Boundaries* (pp 125–136). Boca Raton, FL: CRC Press.

Sujan, M., Spurgeon, P., & Cooke, M. (2015a). The role of dynamic trade-offs in creating safety — A qualitative study of handover across care boundaries in emergency care. *Reliability Engineering & System Safety*, 141, 54–62.

Sujan, M., Spurgeon, P., & Cooke, M. (2015b). Translating tensions into safe practices through dynamic trade-offs: The secret second handover. In R. Wears, E. Hollnagel, & J. Braithwaite (Eds.), *Resilient Health Care, Volume 2: The Resilience of Everday Clinical Work* (pp. 11–22). Farnham, UK: Asghate Publishing.

Vygotsky, L. S. (1978). *Mind in Society*: Cambridge, MA: Harvard University Press.

11 Muddling Through the Built Environment to Preserve Patient Safety and Well-Being

Natália Ransolin, Tarcisio Abreu Saurin and Carlos Torres Formoso

CONTENTS

INTRODUCTION

The built environment (BE) is a key technical dimension of health care services, encompassing the physical spaces, equipment, layout and furniture that support the functions performed by caregivers and patients. As such, the BE design in health care facilities must account for requirements from several stakeholders (Kim, Kim, Cha, & Fischer, 2015). Requirements refer to conditions that express, qualitatively or quantitatively, the properties that a building must have in order to meet stakeholders' needs (Kamara, Anumba, & Evbuomwan, 1999). In health care, the main stakeholder is the patient, whose requirements are intertwined with the requirements of caregivers (Tzortzopoulos, Codinhoto, Kagioglou, Rooke, & Koskela, 2009).

Therefore, understanding the functions performed in health care services is necessary for identifying requirements and their corresponding association with the BE. Functions, which correspond to the activities for producing a required activity, encompass three types (Hollnagel, 2012): technical (e.g., provision of air conditioning in a ward); organisational (e.g., designing an expansion of a hospital unit); or individual (e.g., administering drugs to a patient).

In the context of resilient health care, the Functional Resonance Analysis Method (FRAM) has been used for functional modelling, as it sheds light on performance to cope with the gap between Work-as-Imagined and Work-as-Done. Resilient performance implies filling in gaps in Work-as-Imagined and adapting to variability, such as that arising from unfulfilled BE requirements. In turn, the BE is known to influence patient safety and well-being (PSW) (Zhang, Tzortzopoulos, & Kagioglou, 2018), which is possibly the most fundamental requirement in health care (*"first do not harm"*). In spite of that, the mechanisms linking BE to PSW have not been modelled by previous studies. In this chapter, FRAM is adopted for that purpose, by modelling how the fulfilment (or not) of BE requirements influences functions and then PSW.

In FRAM, a function is described by six aspects: input, output, resources, preconditions, control and time (Hollnagel, 2012). The precondition aspect is particularly relevant for the proposed approach, as it accounts for conditions that must exist before carrying out a function. While a precondition does not start a function, it should be in place before that (Hollnagel, 2012). Therefore, BE requirements can be considered as a type of precondition, creating the possibility of considering those requirements when developing a FRAM model (Ransolin, Saurin, & Formoso, 2020a). Hereafter in this chapter, the terms 'precondition' and 'BE requirements' are used indistinctly, due to the similar role they play in FRAM modelling.

The utility and applicability of this approach were tested in an empirical study in an adult intensive care unit (ICU). A scenario of functional resonance is discussed, highlighting its implications to PSW and resilient health care. Functional resonance is the detectable signal (e.g., an adverse event) that emerges from the unintended interaction of the everyday variability of multiple functions (Hollnagel, 2012).

The study reported in this chapter is part of a broader research project carried out at the same ICU, in which a framework for the integrated modelling of the BE and other functional requirements was applied, by combining the use of FRAM and Building Information Modelling for requirements management (Ransolin et al., 2020a). In a previous paper, Ransolin et al. (2020b) discuss another scenario of functional resonance at the same ICU, using an approach similar to that presented in this chapter.

BUILT ENVIRONMENT IN INTENSIVE CARE UNITS

ICUs are often highly physically and psychologically stressful environments for patients, their families and caregivers (Intensive Care Society, 2016; La Calle, Martin, & Nin, 2017). Common contributing factors to that are noise stimuli, bright lights, room temperature, lack of access to the external environment, lack of privacy and frequent interruptions (La Calle et al., 2017; Pickup, Lang, Atkinson, & Sharples, 2018). Also, the constant presence of light and the resulting loss of awareness of day and night contributes to the condition of delirium in ICU patients, which is a brain dysfunction leading to altered wakefulness and cognition (Fontaine, Briggs, & Pope-Smith, 2001). Another undesired consequence of such an unpleasant environment might be the use of higher medication dosages to cope with discomfort (Rashid, 2010).

Although there are several BE requirements relevant to ICUs, there is scarce litera-ture on which requirements are the most important as well as on design solutions that fulfil those requirements. For example, Valentin and Ferdinande (2011) set out a requirement that 'patient transport to and from the ICU should ideally be separated from public corridors and visitor waiting areas, to ensure patient privacy and fast and unobstructed patient transport'. According to Rashid (2015) another relevant require-ment is that 'the size of an ICU must be appropriate for constant visibility between ICU patients and care providers'. However, quantitative studies have identified weak links between the fulfilment of those requirements and occupants' comfort and satisfaction, which may be due to the difficulty in isolating the impact of the BE (Zhang et al., 2018).

ICUs have also been a setting of interest in resilient health care studies. For exam-ple, Paries et al. (2013) investigated the merger of two separate ICU services, describ-ing how resilience contributed to the improved performance of the new unit. Horsley et al. (2019) presented a framework for the improvement of ICU team resilience. However, relationships with BE issues have not been explored, even though these could be relevant – e.g., ward rounds that support team resilience need to occur in a workspace that accommodates all participants.

RESEARCH METHOD

SCENARIO

This study was carried out in a 34-bed adult ICU, which is part of a major teaching hospital in Southern Brazil. ICU staff is comprised of about 200 employees from 15 professional categories, mostly doctors ($n = 40$), nurses ($n = 32$) and nurse techni-cians ($n = 115$).

The ICU is located on the 13th floor of a 13-floor building. It has two adjacent pods: (i) an older area (21 beds) not originally built to host an ICU, where the bays have on average 9 m^2 and are divided by curtains – this area has a few sinks for hand hygiene and is intended to receive patients with length of stay shorter than 13 days; and (ii) a newer area (13 beds) originally intended to be an ICU, where bays have from 10 to 13 m^2 and are divided by glass walls. Patients admitted to this last pod have a more critical condition and are expected to stay for more than 13 days.

Patients are admitted from the emergency department on the ground floor; the surgical unit on the sixth floor, the wards located on several floors and from other hospitals. Several other areas of the hospital interact with the ICU, involving flow of supplies and staff – e.g., warehouse, radiology, kitchen and central pharmacy.

DATA COLLECTION

The development of the FRAM model was based on the researcher's immersion in the context of the study, which provided opportunities for understanding Work-as-Done as well as for the identification of BE requirements. There were three main sources of data: interviews, observation of functions and analysis of regulations. As for interviews, these involved 24 professionals, 2 members of patient families and 1 patient – who was interviewed after being discharged from the ICU. A script of 12 questions guided the interviews (e.g., how does the BE facilitate or hinder the development of your daily activities?), focussing on the functions performed by the interviewees and the relationships of those functions with the BE.

At least one representative from each main group of stakeholders was interviewed and had their functions observed, including managers – chief administrative, medical and nursing heads; assistance team – doctors, nurses, nurse and radiology technicians, allied health professionals, such as physiotherapist, nutritionist, speech therapist, clinical pharmacist; cleaning team, secretary; patients and their families. In turn, two Brazilian regulations were also analysed: one of them addressed the functioning of health care services (ANVISA, 2010), and the other set out requirements to the BE in hospitals (ANVISA, 2002). Altogether, data collection took 85 hours, being 62 hours for interviews and 23 hours for observations, during 15 visits. The research project was approved by the hospital's ethical committee.

DATA ANALYSIS

Data from the aforementioned sources were subject to a thematic analysis with predefined themes associated with the information needed for developing a FRAM model that could represent the ICU everyday functioning. The themes were: functions; their aspects (input – I, output – O, precondition – P, resources – R, control – C and time – T); and output variability. As mentioned above, all BE requirements were regarded as a type of precondition aspect of functions.

Based on this information, the research team devised the first version of the FRAM model. A key assumption of this model was that there would be two functions defining the model boundaries: <fulfil BE requirements>, which provided preconditions and other aspects to the functions carried out by caregivers; and <receive or respond to care interventions>, which was performed by patients. Variability of the output of this latter function was interpreted as detrimental to PSW.

This draft of the FRAM model was then discussed in 11 face-to-face meetings with doctors, physiotherapist, nurses and nurse technicians. After a final model was produced, researchers and professionals jointly identified possible scenarios of functional resonance that met two criteria: there should be risks to PSW, and the unfulfilment of BE requirements should be a contributing factor to those risks. One of these scenarios is presented in this chapter. It is worth noting that this functional resonance scenario is based on the generic FRAM model, but slightly different from it. The main difference relates to the inclusion of functions that display resilient performance in action – i.e., functions that only existed because resilience was necessary to cope with unfulfilled BE requirements. Although these functions played a key moderating role between the BE and PSW, all those functions in-between <fulfil BE requirements> and <receive or respond to care interventions> were also moderators.

RESULTS

Figure 11.1 presents the functional resonance scenario derived from the overall ICU model. The two previously mentioned functions that set the limits to the model are represented at the bottom and at the top of Figure 11.1. There are six functions

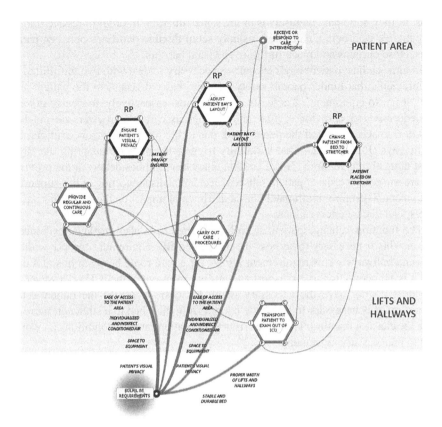

FIGURE 11.1 Functional resonance scenario: influence of the BE on PSW

Notes: (i) waves inside the hexagons and rectangles indicate output variability; (ii) RP next to the hexagons represents functions that display resilient performance.

in-between these two, playing a moderating role. These functions are carried out in two areas: patient bay, and lifts and hallways. These areas are highlighted in the background of Figure 11.1, which also highlights the couplings between <fulfil BE requirements> and the other functions.

The assumption of this scenario is that there was variability of the output of <fulfil BE requirements> – i.e., BE requirements were not fulfilled.

As a result, three functions that displayed resilient performance were triggered, namely: <ensure patient's privacy>, <adjust patient bay's layout> and <change patient from bed to stretcher>. The output of <fulfil BE requirements>, which was not produced, is coupled to the input of those three functions (see Figure 11.1). Although that output is not what starts the resilient functions in everyday work, it is coupled to them as an input in order to convey that resilient performance was necessary only because of unfulfilled BE requirements.

Regarding <ensure patient's privacy>, it arises from the unfulfilled BE requirement 'patient's visual privacy'. According to reports from caregivers, invasive interventions like tracheostomy, scare family members and patients from neighbouring beds, as they anticipate themselves in the same situation. In order to reduce impacts on patient's well-being, caregivers usually setup flexible partitions between patient bays, close curtains and place furniture as visual barriers.

In turn, <adjust patient bay's layout> is necessary to deal with two unfulfilled BE requirements that hinder patient safety, namely 'ease of access to the patient area' and 'space to equipment'. These are requirements, respectively, to <carry out care procedures> and <provide regular and continuous care>. Caregivers do not have 360-degree access around the patient bed, due to the tight and narrow configuration of the bays (Figure 11.2). That variability triggers the need for adapting the bay in most clinical interventions. However, that adaptation implies delays in the provision of care and creates risks of patient falls and accidental disconnection of life-supporting equipment. Therefore, it ultimately has a detrimental impact on the function <receive or respond to care interventions>.

The function <change patient from bed to stretcher> also displays resilience in action. This is necessary to address the unfulfilled BE requirement 'proper width of lifts and hallways'. This requirement allows for a safe route between hospital units and it is a precondition to <transport patient for exams out of the ICU>. However, the elevators do not have the necessary width for easy access of the patient's bed. Therefore, it is necessary to move the patient from their bed to a stretcher, narrower than the elevator opening. This poses risks to the patient, whose condition can worsen due to unnecessary movements.

The outputs of the three resilient functions provided the precondition aspect for three other functions directly related to patient care (see Figure 11.1). Certainly, these preconditions should have been ideally fulfilled as a result of effective BE design. The three care functions that benefitted from resilient performance were:

(i)   <provide regular and continuous care>, which represents every day care provided by the attending nurses;

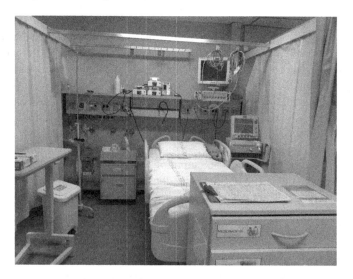

FIGURE 11.2   Patient bay at the ICU (Courtesy of Natália Ransolin)

(ii)   <carry out care procedures>, which involves more specific and technically complicated care activities, such as insertion of intravenous catheters, haemodialysis and mechanical ventilation; and

(iii)   <transport patient to exams out of the ICU>, which may involve, for example, patient transportation from the 13th floor to the radiology unit on the ground floor.

In spite of the aforementioned examples, not all unfulfilled BE requirements are compensated by resilience. This point can be illustrated by the requirement 'individualised and indirect conditioned air in the bays'. At the ICU, there is only one air exit above each bed, from a central air conditioning system that does not allow for customised air temperature in each bay. The absence of compensatory resilience means that the output variability of <fulfil BE requirements> travels unchecked from that function to <receive or respond to care intervention>, thus posing risks to PSW. Overall, in the described scenario, functional resonance accounts for the occurrence of all variabilities associated with unfulfilled BE requirements, partially or totally overlapping in time and space. Their aggregate effect on PSW is expected to be detrimental.

DISCUSSION

Two out of the three functions that displayed resilient performance (i.e., <adjust patient bay's layout> and <ensure patient's visual privacy>) implied small changes in the BE, which had not been anticipated by design. These changes can be interpreted as 'successive limited comparisons' or 'muddling through' (Lindblom, 1959) as they involve performance adjustment on the spot to cope with suboptimal conditions, without following any clear plan. As people gain experience, these adjustments tend to be incrementally more effective over time (Lindblom, 1959). In this way, muddling through has been used in this chapter as a synonym of functions that display resilient performance.

Suboptimal conditions related to BE might be long-lasting and costly to change, therefore offering opportunities for successive limited comparisons on a daily basis. Indeed, the oldest pod at the ICU was built around 50 years ago and some of its original drawbacks persist up to this day, such as the small areas for the bays (see Figure 11.2). Despite risks such as disconnection of life-saving equipment when providing care, researchers were not aware of any adverse event arising from these, which may be an indication of successfully muddling through. It follows from this that functions related to adjustments in the BE possibly reduce detrimental impacts on PSW. As a drawback, these functions introduce additional complexity in the system, by creating new interactions and their own unintended consequences.

The proposed approach could also be useful for modelling how the consequences of muddling through at one level impacts other levels, either immediately or with some delay. A hypothetical example could be related to the muddling through that occurs during the BE design stage of health care facilities, which impacts professionals at the sharp end of health care services. In fact, BE designers muddle through as a result of incomplete information on users' needs, besides being subject to time and financial pressures that hinder users' involvement in the design process (Hicks, McGovern, Prior, & Smith., 2015). All of these interactions (or the absence of needed interactions) across levels might be modelled through FRAM, as suggested by applications to similar purposes in other industries (e.g., Patriarca, Bergström, & Di Gravio, 2017).

CONCLUSION

This chapter has presented a new use for FRAM, namely as an approach for the modelling of how the BE influences patient safety and well-being. Results from the ICU study indicated that FRAM: (i) allowed for mapping BE requirements into functions and (ii) shed light on functions performed by care teams that moderated BE impacts on patient safety and well-being. These functions corresponded to muddling through in a BE context and they were necessary to cope with unfulfilled BE requirements.

Regarding further studies, these could place a greater emphasis on understanding the nature of the functions that display resilient performance, so as to shed light on the extent to which they are unavoidable as well as their unintended consequences. A hypothesis to be empirically investigated is that detrimental effects of suboptimal BE on PSW tend to be lower when there are moderating functions playing a resilient role. Results from these studies may inform a revision of existing methods for the design of health care facilities, which could be based on more realistic assumptions on the nature of the functions performed in these environments.

REFERENCES

Anvisa – Agência Nacional de Vigilância Sanitária. (2002). Resolução de Diretoria Colegiada – *RDC N.50*.
Anvisa – Agência Nacional de Vigilância Sanitária. (2010). Resolução de Diretoria Colegiada – *RDC N.7*.
Fontaine, D. K., Briggs, L. P., & Pope-Smith, B. (2001). Designing humanistic critical care environments. *Critical Care Nursing Quarterly*, 24(3), 21–34.
Hicks, C., McGovern, T., Prior, G., & Smith, I. (2015). Applying lean principles to the design of healthcare facilities. *International Journal of Production Economics*, 170, 677–686.
Hollnagel, E. (2012). *FRAM: The Functional Resonance Analysis Method: Modelling Complex Socio-technical Systems*. Farnham, UK: Ashgate Publishing.
Horsley, C., Hocking, C., Julian, K., Culverwell, P., & Zijdel, H. (2019). Team resilience. In E. Hollnagel, J. Braithwaite, R. Wears (Eds.), *Resilient Health Care, Volume 4: Delivering Resilient Health Ccare* (pp. 97–117). Abingdon, Oxon: Routledge.
Intensive Care Society. (2016). *Guidelines for the Provision of Intensive Care Services*. London, UK: Intensive Care Society. Retrieved September 7 2020, from https://www.ficm.ac.uk/sites/default/files/gpics_ed.1.1_-_2016_-_final_with_covers.pdf.
Kamara, J. M., Anumba, C. J., & Evbuomwan, N. F. (1999). Client requirements processing in construction: A new approach using QFD. *Journal of Architectural Engineering*, 5(1), 8–15.
Kim, T. W., Kim, Y., Cha, S. H., & Fischer, M. (2015). Automated updating of space design requirements connecting user activities and space types. *Automation in Construction*, 50, 102–110.
La Calle, G. H., Martin, M. C., & Nin, N. (2017). Seeking to humanize intensive care. *Revista Brasileira de terapia intensiva*, 29(1), 9–13.
Lindblom, C. E. (1959). The science of "muddling through". *Public Administration Review*, 19(2), 79–88.

Paries, J., Lot, N., Rome, F., & Tassaux, D. (2013). Resilience in intensive care units: The HUG case. In E. Hollnagel, J. Braithwaite, R. Wears (Eds.), *Resilient Health Care.* (pp. 77–96). Farnham, UK: Ashgate Publishing.

Patriarca, R., Bergström, J., & Di Gravio, G. (2017). Defining the functional resonance analysis space: Combining Abstraction Hierarchy and FRAM. *Reliability Engineering and System Safety*, 165, 34–46.

Pickup, L., Lang, A., Atkinson, S., & Sharples, S. (2018). The dichotomy of the application of a systems approach in UK healthcare the challenges and priorities for implementation. *Ergonomics*, 61(1), 15–25.

Ransolin, N., Saurin, T.A., & Formoso, C.T. (2020a). Integrated modelling of built environment and functional requirements: Implications for resilience. *Applied Ergonomics*, 88, 103154.

Ransolin, N., Saurin, T.A., & Formoso, C.T. (2020b). The influence of the built environment on patient safety and wellbeing: A functional perspective. In I. D. Tommelein & E. Daniel (Eds.), *Proceedings of the 28th Annual Conference of the International Group for Lean Construction (IGLC28)*, Berkeley, CA: The International Group for Lean Construction. Retrieved 7 September 2020, from http://iglc.net/Papers/Conference/30.

Rashid, M. (2010). Environmental design for patient families in intensive care units. *Journal of Healthcare Engineering*, 1(3), 367–398.

Rashid, M. (2015). Research on nursing unit layouts: An integrative review. *Facilities*, 33(9/10), 631–695.

Tzortzopoulos, P., Codinhoto, R., Kagioglou, M., Rooke, J. A., & Koskela, L. J. (2009). The gaps between healthcare service and building design: A state of the art review. *Ambiente Construído*, 9(2), 47–55.

Valentin, A., Ferdinande, P., & ESICM Working Group on Quality Improvement. (2011). Recommendations on basic requirements for intensive care units: Structural and organizational aspects. *Intensive Care Medicine*, 37(10), 1575.

Zhang, Y., Tzortzopoulos, P., & Kagioglou, M. (2018). Healing built-environment effects on health outcomes: Environment–occupant–health framework. *Building Research and Information*, 47(6), 747–766.

Part IV

Muddling with Application
In and Around Hospitals

MUDDLING WITH APPLICATION: IN AND AROUND HOSPITALS

The fourth section of the book presents a further four studies which look at the work presented through a 'muddling with purpose' frame. Patterson and Deutsch, international experts in simulation and resilience from the United States of America, discuss their work using in situ simulation which they harness to identify obstacles, shortcomings, solutions and learnings without creating additional risks to patients. This is the benefit of simulation, according to Patterson and Deutsch, and it helps create adaptive capacity which is highly needed when clinicians are faced with both normal and unexpected occurrences in the workplace.

Moving from the micro of the on-the-ground simulation to the macro of big data, de Vos and Hamming from the Netherlands, working at the intersection of Safety-I and Safety-II, look at how patient-level data can be linked to hospital data to shine a light on circumstances where safety is present. This contrasts to the typical stance of researchers in patient safety, who look at where it has been absent.

Several years ago Kitamura and Nakajima from Japan became interested in how patients interact and affirm each other (also called peer-to-peer sharing). Focussed on kidney disease in a Japanese hospital, they document ways the clinicians and hospital staff supported such peer-to-peer information-sharing through a World Café approach, a useful mechanism for encouraging the cross-fertilisation of ideas. This helped patients feel, and actually be, supported as they overcame hurdles and created a better path to meet their own health goals.

Finally, rounding out this section of the book, O'Hara, Baxter and Murray examined the muddling phenomenon through a consideration of research they have been doing with patients and families in transition from hospital to other locations, particularly home. While in traditional health systems this has been seen as a simple problem of providing a discharge summary to patients moving from one setting to another, these United Kingdom authors tease out multiple complex challenges and stress the importance of involving patients and families in such transitional episodes (Figure 1).

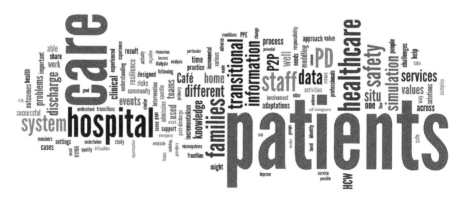

FIGURE 1 A word cloud of Part IV. (Source: http://www.wordle.net/)

12 Simulation to Surface Adaptive Capacity

Mary Patterson and Ellen S. Deutsch

CONTENTS

INTRODUCTION

Frontline health care workers (HCWs) have deep knowledge of the environments in which they work yet their knowledge of their clinical environment as a system, or of the interdependencies of their system with other systems are inevitably incomplete. Similarly, administrative HCWs may have deep knowledge of financial or operational systems, but an inevitably incomplete understanding of frontline patient care delivery. The frontline HCW's ability to care for patients often relies on informal workarounds and adaptations to constantly changing demands and resources. In effect, HCWs 'muddle through' in the best sense of the term (Lindblom, 1959, 1979; Rothmayr Allison & Saint-Martin, 2011). Muddling through and the concept of incomplete knowledge, distributed decision-making and incremental change reflects how microsystems, whether clinical or administrative units, perform work. Work-as-Done (Hollnagel, Wears, & Braithwaite, 2015) often involves '"partisan mutual adjustment", i.e., a process of negotiation and bargaining where decision-makers make compromises and adjust to one another' (Rothmayr Allison & Saint-Martin, 2011) as well as to the changing demands of the work. The way in which this occurs may be unconscious, embedded in tradition or culture. It may be passed from one generation of HCW to the next as a component of the 'hidden curriculum' (Coakley, O'Leary, & Bennett, 2019; Marte, 2019) in a particular microsystem. The culture in much of frontline health care delivery values expertise in overcoming obstacles to get the job done for the current patient (Tucker, 2009). The way in which frontline HCWs muddle through to take care of their patients may be unknown to those HCWs who make high-level decisions about resource allocation (e.g., staffing, equipment) distant from the frontline; and vice versa.

One might ask, if muddling through works for those at the frontline, is there a necessity to study or evaluate it? The reality is that while frontline HCWs may have developed local solutions to a particular challenge, the solution may not be optimal. It may in fact rely on an unsustainable workload and be constrained by inadequate or diminishing resources. Or, a 'first order' adaptation in one microsystem may negatively impact other systems (Tucker, 2009). In some cases, the frontline HCW no longer sees the adaptation as unusual or worthy of note; in other cases, the frontline HCW may believe that a process violation is necessary but may also have concerns that exposing the violation may have repercussions impacting their own employment. Either circumstance, of unrecognised or unreported adaptations, fails to take advantage of opportunities (Deutsch, 2017) to learn or to situate the adaptation in a larger health care system context.

At a higher level, the organisational leadership may not be aware of the degree of adaptation that is occurring and how hard the frontline HCW team is working to care for patients (The Tragedy of Adaptability) (Wears & Hettinger, 2014). In fact, the microsystem may be so stretched that some level of failure is inevitable – whether it occurs by graceful degradation or in a catastrophic manner. From the 'muddling' perspective of incremental change, (Lindblom, 1959, 1979; Rothmayr Allison & Saint-Martin, 2011) surfacing the adaptations which have been implemented allows successive comparison of trade-offs related to patient care values, resources and needs.

WHERE IN SITU SIMULATION FITS IN

Simulation that occurs in the clinical environment provides a method to understand the challenges of daily work by exposing the ambiguous information, shifting workload, time pressure, resource limitations and regulatory constraints as well as the adaptations that frontline HCWs are using.

The structure of in situ simulation, that it occurs in the clinical work environment, often uses available equipment and supplies, and includes many of the disciplines that typically work in such a setting, facilitates understanding of system function as well as system constraints and even the adaptations that various disciplines within the system use to get work done. Initially the knowledge, expertise and limitations of various disciplines may be unknown to other disciplines. The debriefing that follows in situ simulation illuminates both the expertise and limitations of the HCWs as well as the resources and limitations of the system in which they function. For many HCWs, in situ simulation and the debriefing associated with it may be the only time that they think about health care as a distributed complex system with assets, interdependencies and limitations. This multidisciplinary interaction invites reflection on daily work and enables HCWs to identify and address hazards and risks without the psychological burden that accompanies discussions that have a similar intent but occur only after an adverse patient event. This process also invites the development and testing of collaborative solutions to identified threats.

Simulations designed to improve health care delivery processes often demonstrate incremental adaptations, even if muddling was not the recognised or articulated intent. Muddling is implied but not articulated in 'plan – do – study – act' iterative approaches to improvements. For example, a multidisciplinary team of providers participated in simulations to practise the management of post-partum haemorrhage (maternal bleeding after delivery), an uncommon but potentially fatal emergency. During debriefings following the first few simulations, participants identified a number of items that were needed to care for the simulated mother, including equipment, intravenous (IV) fluids, and other medications, some of which were quite specialised for this unique condition. Acquiring these items rapidly was challenging because the items were stored in a variety of locations, such that aggregating all the necessary items was time-consuming. The groups decided to identify specific needed items and locate them together on an emergency cart so that the items could be more rapidly acquired if needed in an emergency. Over the course of several simulations, multiple items were added to the cart, in an incremental manner. However, after a while the cart contained so many items that retrieval of specific items within the cart became cumbersome. The groups made further improvements by identifying some items as easily available even without being stocked in the cart, so those items were selectively removed to achieve the best balance possible at the time. Then the groups decided that the cart might be useful for other emergencies and made further adjustments. With changes in technology, medications and health care practices, it's likely that the contents of the cart will continue to evolve over time.

Another example of the use of in situ simulation to promote adaptation is described in the response to a precursor event (near miss). A paediatric patient presented to a paediatric emergency department with partial airway obstruction from an aspirated foreign body (Johnson, et al., 2012). Though a critical airway management process existed for this situation, this type of event occurred infrequently, and the process did not work as planned. The patient was not harmed, but this was viewed as a risk to other patients given the likelihood that another paediatric patient could have a similar issue. The emergency department, otolaryngology and anaesthesia teams used in situ simulation to test responses in the existing system. They identified that two of six simulated patients would likely have died due to prolonged response times and lack of needed equipment. Working collaboratively, the three groups modified the critical airway response process as well as the means by which equipment was made available emergently. When the new system was tested with in situ simulation, no patient of the six simulated patients died. The process relied on collaboration and negotiation by members of different disciplines. In situ simulation provided a means to identify and test risks as well as test the proposed solutions. This proactive and incremental approach provided a solution at a local level to satisfy the overarching goal of caring for an infrequent but high-risk patient condition (Johnson et al., 2012).

ADAPTATIONS, PANDEMICS AND SIMULATION

As in situ simulation can be used to address near misses, in situ simulation can also address potential hazards. As we write this, the novel coronavirus is spreading globally. Some years ago, the Ebola virus, already raging in West Africa, was perceived to pose a threat to Western countries as well. The perceived threat created urgency for Western health care organisations to develop and test plans to isolate and manage suspected Ebola patients while protecting HCWs; many used simulation to develop and refine those plans. Though most health care organisations had some type of infection control plan, the challenges of managing patients with this virus in a typical health care setting were unprecedented and largely unrecognised. In situ simulations performed to optimise both patient and HCW safety identified challenges and risks that were not appreciated and resulted in adaptations of existing plans that were then tested again with in situ simulations.

The Ebola outbreak was a novel and dynamic situation for most HCWs. The information on recommended levels of personal protection evolved daily. It also became clear as the simulations were performed, that work as typically done would not succeed in this situation. Challenges related to the proper donning and doffing of personal protective equipment (PPE) were unexpected but became starkly apparent during simulations. The proper donning and doffing of PPE required a higher level of training and expertise than typical HCWs possessed. It was observed that housekeeping and security personnel were at particularly high risk especially given the lack of PPE training typically provided to these groups.

The challenges associated with wearing high-level PPE while performing patient care resulted in adaptations to many patient care processes. For example, it became clear that conventional IV or central line placement for medication infusions would be impossible while wearing high-level PPE, thus the decision was made to use intraosseous (IO) lines only. Likewise, it was deemed too dangerous to transport laboratory samples to the main hospital laboratory so only point-of-care testing was performed. Physicians already caring for infected patients were taught to take chest X-rays to minimise the number of additional people exposed to patient secretions. Each of these solutions emerged during in situ simulations as the challenge of preventing HCW exposure was recognised. This episode truly represented muddling through, that is incremental modifications based on the input of frontline HCWs, infectious disease experts and administrative HCWs in the face of ambiguous and incomplete information (Biddell et al., 2016; Phrampus et al., 2016).

The application of similar in situ simulation processes to help with incremental improvements during the novel coronavirus outbreak are obvious, and organisations are now conducting simulations to optimise isolation and management processes for novel coronavirus patients while protecting HCWs. While there were many lessons learned in developing infection prevention and control during the Ebola virus threat, additional considerations, such as grossly insufficient supplies of PPE, have resulted in a need to further modify protocols.

Simulation may also change the way that various disciplines and members of a health care team relate to one another. This also contributes to incremental change in team processes. In this case, the change may occur organically as a result of discussion between formerly siloed groups. For example, a simulation focussed on a paediatric patient with an obstructed tracheostomy was conducted with several multidisciplinary ad hoc teams in a children's hospital. The debriefing revealed that the understanding of physicians and nurses around this particular challenge and the expertise of each role were segregated. Nurses, who often managed routine care and tracheostomy emergencies on the ward, were surprised that not all physicians possessed this knowledge. Physicians were surprised that nurses with the knowledge to manage a tracheostomy emergency hesitated to act and awaited orders from the physician. Although this is one example, it is often observed that the debriefing discussion facilitates the emergence and sharing of previously unknown information between individuals from different roles, and this improved understanding may also enhance their appreciation for each other. In a sense, physicians and nurses were muddling through within their own silos. Psychological safety, a key element of debriefing, encourages sharing of information between members of different disciplines that may not have other opportunities to interact in this way. The debriefing also provides opportunities to develop means of communicating that enable HCWs to quickly share knowledge and expertise with one another and recognise and fill in collective information gaps (e.g., identifying the closest location of replacement tracheostomy tubes). This facilitates a collaborative approach that brings together participants and observers who can contribute a range of information, expertise and resources to address the common challenge.

ON SYSTEMS AND MICROSYSTEMS

On a systems level, in situ simulation enhances the understanding of the ways that various teams approach similar challenges. Simulation allows us to see how different individuals and teams respond to and manage the similar events. Rather than identifying a single 'best' approach to disruptions, in situ simulation often identifies poor design, system and resource issues. It also provides opportunities for the participants to develop solutions. In this situation, incremental changes may be advantageous or problematic. Repeating similar simulation scenarios with different teams may surface common themes about concerns and about potential solutions (Dekker, 2006). In this situation, conducting similar simulations with different teams is consistent with the concept of collaborating and developing incremental change.

Though in situ simulation is often implemented in a single microsystem, it can be used to address a common challenge across a health care organisation or system. Again, the emergence of COVID-19 has demanded improvisation and adaptation by individual HCWs, teams, microsystems and macrosystems. In the early weeks of the COVID-19 pandemic in the United States, there was incomplete information on the best strategies for caring for these patients and for protecting frontline HCWs. In addition, there were inadequate supplies of PPE. This combination of factors led to improvisation and wide variations in practice across the health care organisation. For example, although N95 masks, hoods and Powered Air-Purifying Respirators (PAPRs) were recommended for use with COVID-19 positive patients, N95 masks and PAPRs were and are in short supply. This led to organisational leadership requiring reuse of N-95 masks even though this was not officially sanctioned by agencies such as the Centers for Disease Control and Prevention. This required adaptation at the macrosystem level – making do in the face of inadequate resources and incomplete information – resulted in a variety of individual and microsystem adaptations.

In one (MP's) organisation, the in situ simulation team conducted COVID-19 response simulations in multiple units (microsystems) across the organisation. There was an opportunity to see successful and less successful adaptations around com-munication, methods of intubating patients safely, modification of PPE as well as methods to don and doff PPE. For example, as the specific PPE items were often mixed and matched based on availability, references for the best way to don and doff PPE (and preserve PPE for reuse) did not exist. Frontline HCWs without hoods or PAPRs took to clipping surgical towels or plastic sheets around their necks. This and the requirement to reuse N-95 masks and face shields required development of evolving guidelines to keep HCWs safe and preserve PPE. Faced with the need to perform endotracheal intubation, known to be a potential source of infectious respi-ratory droplets, various homemade devices were developed. Initially, these were clear plastic boxes in which the patient's head rested and the operator intubated through armholes in the plastic box. While these boxes served the purpose, they were heavy, hard to clean and not adjustable to the operator. These evolved rather quickly into a clear plastic sheet draped over an adjustable Mayo stand or table (Figures 12.1 and 12.2). The in situ simulation team had the opportunity to observe the multiple variations in PPE and to share those that were most successful (i.e., most protective and least likely to result in HCW contamination) between the diverse microsystems. Similarly, the challenges posed by the 'intubation box' were apparent during simulations and the in situ simulation team provided a means to share more successful adaptations between microsystems. These simulations occurred as an

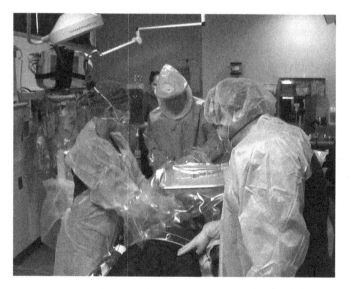

FIGURE 12.1   Intubation of a simulated patient while a portable stand placed above the patient's chest supports a clear plastic drape to contain aerosols emitted from an atomiser adjacent to the patient's mouth. (Courtesy of Mary Patterson)

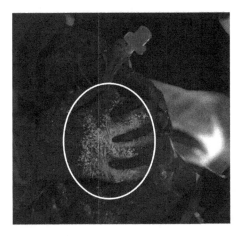

FIGURE 12.2 Simulation demonstrating contamination of HCW's hands grasping manikin's mandible while stabilising an endotracheal tube (projecting from manikin's mouth) during intubation. The circle highlights simulated secretions (Glo Germ Company, Moab, UT), emitted from an atomiser adjacent to the patient's mouth, visualised using ultraviolet light. (Courtesy of Mary Patterson)

iterative process over a period of weeks. The simulation team began to use the simulation planning process with each clinical unit to point out common challenges that would likely need to be addressed. Debriefings were also opportunities to share solutions from other microsystems that had been successful with similar challenges. This did not result in identical solutions but did result in adaptations that were context specific. With virtually all of the organisation's units facing the potential of needing to care for COVID-19 positive patients, in situ simulation provided a means to identify common risks as well as the most successful solutions. Each microsystem did not need to iteratively develop its own solution as the in situ simulation team was able to share information about areas of common risk as well as identify strategies that had already proven successful. This occurred in the face of daily changes of algorithms for testing, patient care and PPE use as well as shifting availability of equipment and PPE.

As in situ simulation teams responded to the COVID-19 pandemic, we developed novel ways of understanding the needs of individual microsystems, but also integrating identified common risks. In this way, the shared risks of microsystems were addressed. Similarly, while it would not have been our usual practice to share solutions identified in other microsystems as potential solutions for a different microsystem, the shared risk and the time pressure made this approach efficient and effective. There were additional incremental gains that were again shared via in situ simulation. While the in situ simulation team was in communication with the organisation's emergency response and infection control leadership, the information and solutions developed were not shared via 'official' communication but rather via oral and written communications between the in situ simulation team and the clinical leaders and educators of various microsystems. In situ simulation served to facilitate non-centralised partisan mutual adjustment and incremental decision-making (Lindblom, 1979) to enable effective adaptations in the context of ambiguous and shifting challenges.

DISCUSSION AND CONCLUSION

In situ simulation can serve as a tool to identify and address common risks and possible solutions across diverse macrosystems even beyond individual organisational boundaries. A simulation-based study by Maa and colleagues explored the administration of epinephrine for simulated anaphylaxis in 28 health care institutions in six countries (Maa et al., 2020). Findings included common errors and latent safety threats as well as conditions associated with fewer errors, thereby providing information that multiple organisations could use to assess and potentially improve their own processes. In this way, in situ simulation enabled a logical approach to understanding risk, but also to identifying the conditions and resources that facilitate good outcomes. This type of deliberate collaboration and spread of in situ simulation holds promise for enhancing capacity in health care systems that collaborate even beyond international borders.

In addition to identifying and mitigating challenges, simulation provides an opportunity to identify factors that contribute to a team's successful performance. This may include identifying specific behaviours, resources, skills and conditions that facilitate good performance. Again, debriefing offers the opportunity to identify the means that various individuals and teams use to adapt to disruptions and what facilitates those adaptations (Dieckmann et al., 2017). There is also the opportunity to understand which adaptations reliably increase the likelihood of good performance. As with our COVID-19 pandemic experiences, in situ simulation can serve to connect and spread successful adaptations. Changes developed through simulation may be seen as 'muddling' because, as knowledge, resources and medical conditions evolve, the perfect immutable solution can never be achieved, but the simulation processes developed to achieve progress are thoughtful and intentional. Perhaps the most profound lesson from simulations comes from reinforcing that the adaptations developed by individuals and teams reflect an underlying adaptive capacity that is valuable and can be nurtured.

REFERENCES

Biddell, E. A., Vandersall, B. L., Bailes, S. A., Estephan, S. A., Ferrara, L. A., Nagy, K. M., … Patterson, M. D. (2016). Use of simulation to gauge preparedness for ebola at a free-standing children's hospital. *Simulation in Healthcare: The Journal of the Society for Medical Simulation*, 11(2), 94–99.
Coakley, N., O'Leary, P., & Bennett, D. (2019). 'Waiting in the wings'; Lived experience at the threshold of clinical practice. *Medical Education*, 53(7), 698–709.
Dekker, S. (2006). *The Field Guide to Understanding Human Error*. Farnham, UK: Ashgate Publishing.
Deutsch, E. S. (2017). Workarounds: Trash or treasure? *Pennsylvania Patient Safety Advisory*, 14(3):1–6.

Dieckmann, P., Patterson, M., Lahlou, S., Mesman, J., Nystrom, P., & Krage, R. (2017). Variation and adaptation: Learning from success in patient safety-oriented simulation training. *Advances in Simulation*, 2(21), 1–14.

Hollnagel, E., Wears, R., & Braithwaite, J. (2015). *From Safety-I to Safety-II: A White Paper*. Resilient Health Care Net: University of Southern Denmark, University of Florida, USA, and Macquarie University, Australia. Retrieved 7 September 2020, from https://resilienthealthcare.net/wp-content/uploads/2018/05/WhitePaperFinal.pdf.

Johnson, K., Geis, G., Oehler, J., Meinzen-Derr, J., Bauer, J., Myer, C., & Kerrey, B. (2012). Simulation to implement a novel system of care for pediatric critical airway obstruction. *Archives of Otolaryngology – Head and Neck Surgery*, 138(10), 907–911.

Lindblom, C. E. (1959). The science of "muddling through". *Public Administration Review*, 19(2), 79–88.

Lindblom, C. E. (1979). Still muddling, not yet through. *Public Administration Review*, 39(6), 517–526.

Maa, T., Scherzer, D. J., Harwayne-Gidansky, I., Capua, T., Kessler, D. O., Trainor, J. L., … Biddell, E. (2020). Prevalence of errors in anaphylaxis in kids (PEAK): A multicenter simulation-based study. *The Journal of Allergy and Clinical Immunology: In Practice*, 8(4), 1239–1246.e3.

Marte, D. (2019). Can a woman of color trust medical education? *Academic Medicine*, 94(7), 928–930.

Phrampus, P. E., O'Donnell, J. M., Farkas, D., Abernethy, D., Brownlee, K., Dongilli, T., & Martin, S. (2016). Rapid development and deployment of Ebola readiness training across an academic health system: The critical role of simulation education, consulting, and systems integration. *Simulation in Healthcare: The Journal of the Society for Medical Simulation*, 11(2), 82–88.

Rothmayr Allison, C., & Saint-Martin, D. (2011). Half a century of "muddling": Are we there yet? *Policy and Society*, 30(1), 1–8.

Tucker, A. L. (2009). *Workarounds and resiliency on the front lines of health care*. Retrieved 7 September 2020, from https://psnet.ahrq.gov/perspective/workarounds-and-resiliency-front-lines-health-care.

Wears, R. L., & Hettinger, A. Z. (2014). The tragedy of adaptability. *Annals of Emergency Medicine*, 63, 338–339.

13 Towards Safety-II in Hospital Care Using the Available Safety-I Environment

Patient-Level Linkage of Currently Available Hospital Data

Marit S. de Vos and Jaap F. Hamming

CONTENTS

CURRENT USE OF PATIENT SAFETY DATA

Most hospitals have more than one system in place to collect data for quality and safety improvement purposes. Staff reporting, record review, mortality and morbidity conferences and patient feedback mechanisms all produce large volumes of data on negative health care outcomes, such as adverse events, incidents or patient complaints. In some settings, it is mandatory to have these data systems in place, and some may even be linked to financial reimbursement. These systems have been installed at different times and for different purposes. As a result, the data often remain isolated from each other and separated from generic registries, such as the database of all in hospital admissions. Although the primary purpose of quality and safety data is to offer a 'window' into the system, these data may currently not be used to their full potential for a more holistic or 'panoramic view' on patient safety. While each system captures different important signals from a patient's journey, using each system individually has some important disadvantages and limitations.

FOCUSSING ON THE NEGATIVE

An important limitation is that these data sources all focus on only the negative outcomes of health care, with analyses often discussing actions that *did not happen*, sometimes referred to as 'failing barriers'. This also introduces a risk of over-simplification, implying, for example, that the negative event could have been prevented if only something specific would have been done (more precisely). This fails to acknowledge many inevitable features of the health care working environment, such as the need for trade-offs between efficiency and thoroughness, and how unexpected outcomes can emerge from combinations of normal courses of actions ('resonance' – an important underlying principle in Safety-II theory). Moreover, regardless of all this uncertainty and complexity, patients are mainly kept safe and why this mostly happens is just as relevant a question as why this sometimes does not.

REAL-WORLD COMPLEXITY AND RELATIONS BETWEEN EVENTS REMAIN OBSCURED

Another missed opportunity lies in the fact that using these data systems in isolation does not allow analysis of how these events may be related at the patient level. To illustrate, incidents or complications can increase a case's complexity and vulnerability, which may trigger more problems.

Linkage of these data sets on the patient level could potentially increase insight into these types of relations between events co-occurring in inpatient admissions. In other words, data linkage may reveal some of the complex relations that are present between events in everyday practice. More specifically, current analyses used in record review or incident reporting only assess one-on-one relations in one direction, that is, from process to subsequent harm. Real clinical practice is more complex, and events within a single admission can have many-to-many relations, which could also be in the opposite direction when initial harm triggers subsequent process problems (e.g., delirium → incident with dislodged intravenous line → haemorrhage → anaemia → transfusion incident).

While currently used in isolation, connecting these different data sources at the patient level would produce one comprehensive dataset that can be used to:

(1) Help reveal the bigger picture of hospital performance, including unsuccessful as well as successful outcomes of everyday work;
(2) Assess these data in relation to each other, offering a perspective that is closer to the messy reality of everyday clinical practice that can be used to trace resilient behaviour and situations in which staff are muddling through with purpose.

CONNECTING THE DATA SILOS

Data from a recently published study can be used to illustrate and discuss implications of patient-level linkage of various sources for safety data in hospitals (de Vos, Hamming, Chua-Hendriks & Marang-van de Mheen, 2019).

MATERIAL AND METHODS

In this study, data from the following registries were linked at the patient level:

- hospital admission registry (generic admission and patient characteristics);
- adverse events registry (embedded in electronic health records);
- incident reporting registry (reported by staff into a hospital-wide system);
- patient complaints' registry (letters archived in binders).

These data have been routinely collected in the surgical department of a Dutch academic hospital between January 2008 and December 2014 for all inpatient admissions. In the Netherlands, adverse event (or complication) registries are used to report patient harm, such as a surgical site infection. By contrast, incident reporting is primarily used to report process problems, i.e., suboptimal situations that (could) cause harm to patients, such as a medication error. More details and definitions can be found in previous publications (de Vos et al., 2019; de Vos, Hamming & Marang-van de Mheen, 2017).

A comprehensive dataset that includes data on inpatient admissions (i.e., patient and admission characteristics) as well as negative events (i.e., incidents, adverse events, patient complaints) can help reveal several aspects of the provided care that would have otherwise remained obscured.

REVEALING THE POSITIVE

In this study, most admissions (78.3% of 26,383) had neither adverse events, nor incidents, nor complaints (Figure 13.1). This could in part have been the result of underreporting, but certainly also reflects how most patients leave the hospital without any problems. Data linkage helps to reveal these cases that otherwise remain obscured, or in other words, helps to visualise 'the other side of the coin'. Usually detection of these cases is a paradoxical 'diagnosis per exclusionem' since there are no dedicated systems to collect cases where 'nothing goes wrong'. To illustrate, the 20,656 cases in this study with neither incidents nor adverse events nor complaints would not be included in any hospital safety database. These cases seem to have left the hospital without any problems, despite 20% being older than 70 years and 70% receiving surgery (of which 28% was emergent and/or with American Society of Anesthesiologists status (ASA) $\geq$ 3) (unpublished numbers).

Similarly, such a comprehensive dataset can be used to study events in relation to each other, such as cases in which process problems occurred but no patient harm or complaints followed. While there were 1,599 cases for which incidents were reported, 54% of these cases had no adverse events. Moreover, for clinicians this

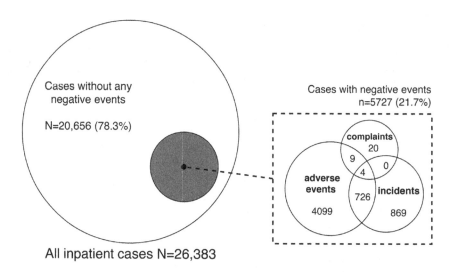

FIGURE 13.1 Overview of all inpatient admissions and occurrence of adverse events, incidents and patient complaints

approach would mean that the data they report during busy everyday clinical practice (e.g., incidents, adverse events) are no longer solely used to focus on 'wrongdoing' but to appreciate how they mostly manage to provide safe and successful care.

TARGET GROUPS

With both positive and non-positive outcomes present within a comprehensive database, cases with increased vulnerability and complexity can be assessed in a more holistic manner. For example, out of 300 inpatient cases receiving emergency surgery with age above 70 years and ASA status ≥ 3, more than one in three cases still had only positive outcomes (i.e., no adverse events, incidents or complaints) in our study. Another example is that while delirium was present among 36% of the 84 cases with patient accidents, there were another 411 patients with delirium without accidents. Again, this can in part be caused by underreporting, but will definitely also be a reflection of enacted resilience by health care professionals, as even high-risk cases with perhaps 'the odds against them' still left the hospital without any problems.

In addition to targeting specific patient groups, integrated data could help to identify and study particularly 'safe' teams or hospital processes in an attempt to understand how they manage to achieve good outcomes, potentially revealing exemplary behaviour and solutions that are already present in the hospital system (similar to the concepts of 'positive deviance' (Lawton, Taylor, Clay-Williams & Braithwaite, 2014) and 'exnovation' (Mesman, 2011)).

REVEALING RESILIENT BEHAVIOUR AND MUDDLING AT THE SHARP END

In commonly used patient safety data analyses, cases with negative events are labelled as 'complicated cases'. For this group, the delivered care was not up to standard. The aftermath of the negative events is not part of the analyses. In everyday clinical practice, however, a lot happens in the aftermath. After all, the emergence of a complication and the accompanying changed conditions of the case require a different response from staff as well as an anticipation of different needs and challenges looking forward. In light of the concept of 'muddling through', this is precisely where we are likely to find decisions made by staff on the spot to fit the situations as it is seen at the moment.

These examples of responding and anticipating are examples of purposefully muddling through. Resilience engineering proposes several abilities necessary for resilient performance (Hollnagel, 2015), including the ability to respond to (ir)regular changes, disturbances and opportunities as well as anticipate potential disruptions, demands or conditions. With this in mind, we could use currently available hospital data to take a closer look at how our staff is acting resilient when negative events arise, attempting to prevent additional problems. To support staff with this process of monitoring and anticipating, hospitals could start by providing a clear overview of all negative events that have been reported for a patient in their electronic medical record. After all, incomplete data and information force people to muddle through, making muddling through not just a convenient solution but also the only solution. Additionally, greater transparency about what is already reported for a specific patient would also help prevent the same incident from being reported more than once, which we frequently came across in this study's data.

CONCLUSION

Patient-level linkage of currently existing quality and safety data in hospitals can help to reveal the bigger picture of patient safety in hospitals by revealing cases in which safety has been *present,* despite ever-present risks and challenges (e.g., high ASA status or elderly patients). This would enable using this currently available 'Safety-I data' for a more holistic, realistic and a Safety-II approach as it enables to also appreciate successful performance by those who reported the data in the first place. Practical implications include using this comprehensive dataset to target certain settings, processes or patient groups for further study of enacted resilience, e.g. where things went well despite certain circumstances or challenges, and how and where staff may be 'muddling through with purpose'.

REFERENCES

de Vos, M.S., Hamming, J. F., Chua-Hendriks, J. J. C., & Marang-van de Mheen, P. J. (2019). Connecting perspectives on quality and safety: Patient-level linkage of incident, adverse event and complaint data. *BMJ Quality and Safety*, 28, 180–189.

de Vos, M. S., Hamming, J. F., & Marang-van de Mheen, P. J. (2017). Learning from morbidity and mortality conferences: Focus and sustainability of lessons for patient care. *Journal of Patient Safety*. [Epublication ahead of print]. 10.1097/PTS.0000000000000440.

Hollnagel, E. (2015). *Introduction to the Resilience Analysis Grid (RAG)*. Retrieved 30 August 2019, from http://erikhollnagel.com/onewebmedia/RAG Outline V2.pdf.

Lawton, R., Taylor, N., Clay-Williams, R., & Braithwaite, J. (2014). Positive deviance: A different approach to achieving patient safety. *BMJ Quality and Safety*, 23, 880–883.

Mesman, J. (2011). Resources of strength: An exnovation of hidden competences to preserve patient safety. In: E. Rowley, & J. Waring (Eds.), *A Sociocultural Perspective on Patient Safety* (pp. 71–92). Surry, UK: Ashgate Publishing.

14 Peer-to-Peer Information Sharing for a High-Quality, Autonomous and Efficient Health Care System

Harumi Kitamura and Kazue Nakajima

CONTENTS

GAPS IN CARE GOALS BETWEEN HEALTH CARE PROVIDERS AND PATIENTS

INCREASING RECOGNITION OF PATIENT ENGAGEMENT AND PATIENT-CENTRED CARE

'Crossing the Quality Chasm' published in 2001 has shed light on patients as important resources that should be actively involved in their own care to improve safety and quality in health care. Patients currently play significant roles to 'keep watch' for their safety. For example, patients have been asked to engage in patient identification (World Health Organization, 2007), confirm results of their x-ray scans (The Royal College of Radiologists, 2016) and speak up to avoid harm (The Joint Commission, 2020). Patient engagement is also recognised as a key component of patient-centred care which requires health care providers to take into consideration the patients' values, preferences and needs in setting care goals. Respect for things that matter to patients is one of the most important indicators of quality and safety from the per-spective of patients (Gerteis, Edgman-Levitan, Daley, & Delbanco, 1993).

Kidney disease is a chronic illness in which patient engagement is important, particularly in the two phases. One is decision-making on which dialysis modality (haemodialysis (HD), peritoneal dialysis (PD), or kidney transplantation) a patient should undergo. The other is life-long self-management of clinical conditions. Both decision-making on a treatment modality and self-management capacity would affect patients' disease prognoses and quality of life. In reality, patients are often forced to muddle through difficulties in their life-long journeys with illness, rather than partici-pating in their own care due to a lack of support for patient engagement in the current health care system.

PROBLEMS IN DECISION-MAKING ON DIALYSIS MODALITY

Patients are not always involved in the decision-making when choosing a dialysis modality nor asked about their values and preferences relating to the treatment. In Japan, the proportion of patients undergoing PD among all patients on dialysis was only 2.8% (Japanese Society for Dialysis Therapy, 2019), which was extremely low compared to 22% in Northern Europe and 7% in the United States (Jain, Blake, Cordy, & Garg, 2012). One reason for the high uptake of HD would be that patients were not provided with sufficient information about PD by their doctors at the pre-dialysis stage. A survey of Japanese dialysis patients ($N = 234$) conducted by an association of patients with kidney diseases in 2008 found that only 39% of patients with HD were involved in making decisions on choosing their dialysis modality. Another survey in 2019 of Japanese dialysis patients ($N = 502$) by a non-profit organ-isation (NPO) of patients with kidney diseases revealed that only 47% of the dialysis patients were given information on both HD and PD and only 38% were asked by their doctors about their preferences or values in decision-making (Japanese NPO of Support for Patients with Kidney Diseases, 2019).

There are several barriers to implementation of patient engagement in decision-making for health care providers: constraints on time and human resources for lengthy interactions with patients and their families; difficulties in understanding patients' life styles; lack of expertise concerning detailed procedures about each dif-ferent dialysis modality. On another front, patients often experience difficulty in anticipating their future life styles with the dialysis modality they choose. Consequently, they tend to choose HD because it is recommended by their doctors, is dominant among the dialysis modality, or appears to be an easier option for patients in terms of self-engagement in care.

Shared decision-making (SDM) as a form of patient engagement can be a key strategy of patient-centred care (Barry, & Edgman-Levitan, 2012; Morton, Tong, Howard, Snelling, & Webster, 2010). Since 2018, Japanese societies for kidney dis-ease have been actively promoting SDM along with the health insurance reimburse-ment scheme for hospitals, providing SDM tools for health care professionals. The new guideline of The International Society for Peritoneal Dialysis (ISPD) in 2020 recommends that goal-directed PD should be prescribed to achieve patients' own life goals based on an individualised SDM approach (Brown et al., 2020). These efforts are expected to accelerate patient engagement in the decision-making process on dialysis modality.

PROBLEMS IN SELF-MANAGEMENT OF LIFE-LONG ILLNESS

Another major challenge in patient engagement is self-management of life-long illness requiring dialysis. Self-management is very important but not so easy for patients, particularly in balancing the control of medical conditions (uremic symptoms, oedema, blood pressure, etc.) and joy in life (meals, bathing, hobbies, etc.). The Standardized Outcomes in Nephrology (SONG)-PD study focussing on the differing care goals between physicians and patients on PD (Manera et al., 2019; SONG-PD Workshop Investigators, 2020) found that physicians often placed importance on evidence and clinical outcomes such as mortality and complications. In contrast, patients undergoing PD place importance on *"the ability to do usual activities."* Another study of patients with HD (Evangelidis et al., 2017) showed similar results that *"Patients gave higher priority to lifestyle-related outcomes."*

Information about how to reconcile such gaps in care goals between patients and health care providers is limited. When a nephrologist warns his or her patient with leg oedema to refrain from eating salty food, the patient would answer 'I have been doing it already' (Joseph-Williams et al., 2017). When patients experience disturbances, e.g., disease progression, changes in jobs or caregivers, their doctors fail to give specific suggestions to patients about how to adapt to the changing environments and how to maintain a sense of normality. Furthermore, patients often find it difficult to continue their usual activities while undergoing dialysis and easily lose hope (as shown at the lowest step in Figure 14.1). Even if patients had chosen PD through SDM and set their own life goals, they would face a gap between the imagined PD life and the real PD life. The information needed by patients to bridge the gap is not written in textbooks nor obtained from their health care providers. One of the major reasons for that is the gaps in care goals between health care providers and patients, as the SONG-PD (Manera et al., 2019; SONG-PD Workshop Investigators, 2020) study revealed.

Fortunately, through conversation with PD patients in clinical practice, we found that patients had unique knowledge to overcome various difficulties based on their own experiences such as practical methods to restrict salt intake while enjoying their daily lives. We hypothesised that sharing patients' experiences with other patients who have the same illness can empower them and increase their self-management capacity balancing both disease and life management. The barrier to sharing patients' knowledge and experiences is that patients usually don't have opportunities to talk with other patients who have, or had overcome, similar adversities. Thus, we planned to hold a World Café style-workshop with PD patients as a peer-to-peer support, called 'PD Café' and examined the effect of the peer support on patients' adaptive capacity.

A WORLD CAFÉ STYLE-WORKSHOP WITH PD PATIENTS

SETTING AND DEVELOPMENT OF THE PD CAFÉ

The setting of the study was the outpatient department for kidney diseases in Osaka University Hospital with 1,086 beds which provides renal replacement therapies,

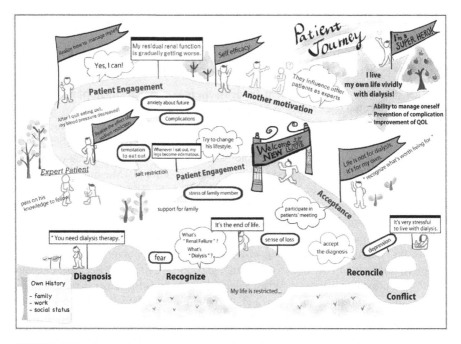

FIGURE 14.1   Patient journey (an example of a patient with end-stage kidney disease)

including HD, PD and kidney transplantation. We provide consultations on dialysis modalities in an SDM setting, and have a high proportion of patients choosing PD. Approximately 35 PD patients are currently followed in the outpatient setting. The age of patients spans 18 to 93 years and the duration of PD ranges from 1 month to 10 years. The department policy is that patients undergoing PD need to consider switching to, or combining with HD when the volume of urine has decreased and becomes less than 200 mL per day.

The departmental PD team including the author (Kitamura), a lead physician, has held an annual meeting for patients undergoing PD since 2008. Although programmes of the meetings have consisted of mainly lectures about PD, some patients expressed their desire to talk with other patients undergoing PD to share information. The style of the meeting changed from a lecture style to a World Café style in 2017 in order to provide a platform for peer-to-peer information sharing (Figure 14.2). The purpose of the PD Café is for patients to share their experience, knowledge and worries with each other in a nurturing space.

THE PROGRAMME AND METHODS OF THE PD CAFÉ

For the purpose of educating patients and families, we have held the annual meeting with the PD Café every year since 2017. Approximately 50 people with various PD experiences, including patients at the pre-dialysis stage, patients who had graduated from PD to HD, and their family members, participated in the PD Café every year. The proportion of family members participating was 30% to 40%. All patients

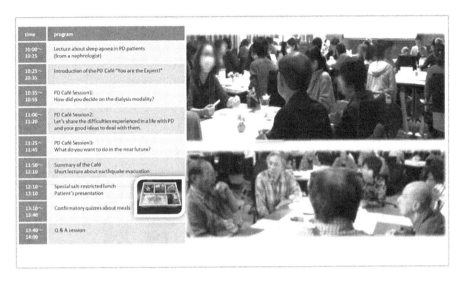

time	program
10:00~ 10:25	Lecture about sleep apnea in PD patients (from a nephrologist)
10:25~ 10:35	Introduction of the PD Café "You are the Expert!"
10:35~ 10:55	PD Café Session1: How did you decide on the dialysis modality?
11:00~ 11:20	PD Café Session2: Let's share the difficulties experienced in a life with PD and your good ideas to deal with them.
11:25~ 11:45	PD Café Session3: What do you want to do in the near future?
11:50~ 12:10	Summary of the Café Short lecture about earthquake evacuation
12:10~ 13:10	Special salt-restricted lunch Patient's presentation
13:10~ 13:40	Confirmatory quizzes about meals
13:40~ 14:00	Q & A session

FIGURE 14.2   World Café for patients undergoing PD (Courtesy of Harumi Kitamura)

undergoing PD or at the pre-dialysis stage who had decided to undergo PD in the outpatient department were notified of the PD Café. The meeting including the PD Café was held on Sunday morning in the large conference room in our hospital. The 2019 programme meeting took four hours. The meeting commenced with a 15-minute physician's lecture about sleep apnoea in PD patients, followed by the PD Café. After the PD Café, participants had a special salt-restricted lunch with the total amount of salt limited to under 2.0 grams, which was arranged by the hospital's dietitian and a chef from a famous Japanese restaurant. During lunch time, one of the patients spontaneously made a 15-minute presentation about his experiences of travelling abroad. After lunch, participants were involved in a 30-minute confirmatory quiz about important points and a 10-minute Q & A session.

With regards to the PD Café, we set up 10 small groups of participants. Each group included four to five patients, family members and a staff member (a dietitian, a nurse of the ward, or a regional liaison office member) as a facilitator. Excluding a PD nurse and a PD doctor from the facilitators, we created an atmosphere where patients were able to talk freely and enjoy peer-to-peer communication. The rules of engagement for the PD Café followed that of the World Café. The participants discussed one topic per session. The three topics were as follows: (1) How did you decide on the dialysis modality?; (2) Let's share the difficulties experienced in a life with PD and your good ideas to deal with them.; (3) What do you want to do in the near future?

As shown in Figure 14.3, after discussing the first topic for 20 minutes, participants moved to different tables, and engaged in another 20-minute discussion with different members, then returned to their original tables. They wrote down comments and ideas they received from other patients on a large piece of paper on each table so they were able to share the information discussed at the table. It was designed to help patients and family members make links with each other, bringing diverse

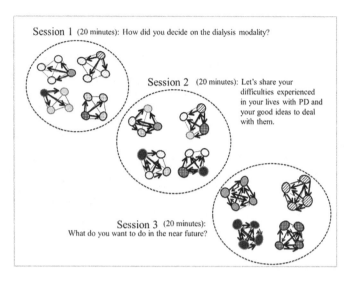

FIGURE 14.3   The rules of the World Café

people together, and building bridges between each patient's original experience. We conducted a questionnaire survey distributed to participants and the staff after each PD Café.

The small circles represent each participant and the arrows indicate interactions between participants. The intensity of the grey colour fill or pattern reflects the amount of information each participant has. In session 1, an experienced patient gave some information to other members at the same table. In session 2, they moved to different tables. They shared the ideas that they obtained in the previous session with new members. In session 3, each member came back to their original table and shared the ideas they had in the previous sessions. As a result, each participant was able to share in all the information provided in the three sessions.

EFFECTS OF PEER-TO-PEER INTERACTIONS

We found five common effects of the PD Café: a sense of connection with other people; motivation for learning; anticipation of their futures; a sense of self-esteem; recognition of value of patients' experience-based knowledge.

First, the peer-to-peer interactions gave patients a sense of connection through empathy. Patients who had faced the same difficulties and tried to overcome them were able to understand each other and became assured. The patients at the pre-dialysis stage, who were in the most physically and mentally stressful and exhausting part of the process, were greatly relieved by the peer-to-peer interactions. All of the PD Café participants answered that they were able to have a sense of connection. After the PD Café session, they said things like:

'I felt a sense of connection among us'.

'I was relieved to know that patients other than myself have the same difficulties in their PD lives'.

'I (patient at pre-dialysis stage) feel very relieved to see and listen to experienced patients. They look so energetic'.

Second, the peer-to-peer interactions motivated them to learn. Each patient already undergoing PD also learnt various ideas including good ways to bathe in a hot spring, travel abroad while undergoing PD, and eat sushi without taking too much salt at the PD Café. Patients at the pre-dialysis stage felt ready to learn about their treatments and the importance of self-management and after experienced relief. As a result, every year, 80–90% of the PD Café participants answered that they were motivated to manage themselves and live actively after the session. They said things like:

'I'd like to travel around the world like that patient!'
'I want to take up playing guitar'.
'I'm going to try cooking with apple cider vinegar instead of soy sauce, which she taught us to decrease the salt intake'.
'I (patient at pre-dialysis stage) learned from other patients that the dialysis is never scary as long as I have the correct knowledge of it'.

Third, the peer-to-peer interactions enabled them to anticipate the future. In peer-to-peer networking, experienced patients shared real experiences and feelings on dialysis, both good and bad, which contributed to closing the gap between 'PD-as-imagined' and 'PD-as-reality'. They could learn the possible path they would take, and how to troubleshoot and strategise for living well with dialysis based on other patients' stories. They learned what they should do when they have abdominal pain, when their urine volume decreases, when they have to switch dialysis modality from PD to HD and so on. According to the survey results, 89% of the participants were able to anticipate and prepare for problems in the future, which may prevent emergent hospitalisations and large fluctuations in the patient's journey.

Fourth, the peer-to-peer interactions gave experienced patients a sense of self-esteem, knowing that they were able to help patients going through a similar process. Approximately 90% of experienced patients said they were happy to tell other people about their original experiences. They answered as follows:

'It is important to pass on my knowledge and experiences to other patients'.
'Painting and giving my advice to others are my passion'.
'To give advice to others is to review my self-management skill'.

The peer-to-peer interactions empowered both experienced and newly diagnosed patients, which may lead to patient autonomy.

Fifth, the peer-to-peer sessions made health care providers realise the value of patients' experience-based knowledge. They were so impressed to see patients at the pre-dialysis stage who had been full of anxiety become positive just after the peer-to-peer interactions. They also realised that patients' experience-based knowledge had much more power than doctor's persuasion to effectively improve patients' self-management skills. Furthermore, they learned the importance of giving individualised practical advice along with each person's circumstances. After the PD Café, young dietitians and nurses said the following:

'For the first time, I learned about the real PD life and noticed what patients felt difficulty in'.

'This Café is useful for us to learn how to give advice in a more effective way'.

'I was so moved and encouraged by the power of patients!'

Not only patients but also health care professionals have been motivated by the peer-to-peer interactions.

As shown in Figure 14.1, experience-based advice from peers promoted patient engagement and improved the skill of self-management. Also, transmitting their original experiences to other patients gave them another value to live with chronic conditions. Like these, an autonomous mutual support system was formed from peer-to-peer networking.

DISCUSSION

One of the challenges that patients suffering from chronic diseases face is to navigate their conditions with limited information given by their doctors. The main care goal for most patients undergoing PD was 'life participation', reflecting their wish for flexibility and autonomy. Although health care professionals prioritised clinical outcomes such as infection and mortality, these 'successes from the medical point of view' were not the most important issues for patients undergoing PD. Such patients need practical information that will help them integrate the treatment into their everyday lives.

If care is compared to mountain climbing, doctors can just say, 'You can go to the top of the mountain only if you climb it'. But a person who climbs a mountain for the first time would face many difficulties trying to successfully reach the top of the mountain. If an experienced climber could share their knowledge with them, they would feel relieved to be able to get plenty of practical, effective advice about which shoes should be worn and how much water should be brought, for instance. They would be able to anticipate some difficulties such as unexpected heavy rain and getting lost, and learn how to respond to them. Therefore, an experienced person's knowledge may enable novices to find a way out of difficulties more efficiently. It is even better if they can get various information from diverse experts.

Likewise, sharing experience-based knowledge among peers through the PD Café seemed much more helpful for patients to increase their capacity for life-long self-management than health care providers' medical book-based advice, according to the results of our study. The study also suggested that patients' experience-based information empowered novice patients to move forward and pursue their life-goals without giving up things that mattered to them. Moreover, peer-to-peer interactions might bring further benefit to pre-dialysis patients in decision-making. Lifestyle-related advice from expert patients could mitigate the anxiety of pre-dialysis patients, help to anticipate their own lifestyles with dialysis and make decisions with assurance. Peer-to-peer interactions in the short-time World Café meeting can be a more powerful approach to facilitate patient engagement not only in life-long self-management but also in decision-making rather than the traditional health care provider-to-patient approach. To develop the peer support system, a convener who provides spaces where people can come together to learn and share experience-based knowledge is needed. Then you just have to let patients 'dance' freely at the PD Café.

For the future development of patient engagement by peer support, we aim to implement the PD Café in other hospitals or for different chronic illnesses. As part of the strategy, we have invited PD care teams from other hospitals to our PD Café so that they can observe the positive influence of peer-to-peer interactions. We are also planning to have a joint Café among neighbouring hospitals, each of which have a small number of PD patients. An online PD Café would provide easier access for patients, especially under the COVID-19 pandemic. We also need to find methods to measure effects of peer support on quality and safety, health outcome and health care cost.

CONCLUSION

Peer-to-peer interactions through the PD Café helped patients to mitigate their anxiety, overcome difficulties related to illness and life, and find their own goals in their life-long journeys. Patients were able to move forward with confidence, anticipating their future lives instead of muddling through. Peer-to-peer networking has the potential to re-design the current health care system by promoting patients' autonomy and changing health care providers' mindset.

REFERENCES

Barry, M. J., & Edgman-Levitan, S. (2012). Shared decision making – Pinnacle of patient-centered care. *New England Journal of Medicine*, 366(9), 780–781.

Brown E. A., Blake, P. G., Boudville, N., Davies, S., de Arteaga, J., Dong, J., … Warady, B. (2020). International Society for Peritoneal Dialysis practice recommendations: Prescribing high-quality goal-directed peritoneal dialysis. *Peritoneal Dialysis International*, 40(3), 244–253.

Evangelidis, N., Tong, A., Manns, B., Hemmelgarn, B., Wheeler, D. C., Tugwell, P., … Sautenet, B. (2017). Developing a set of core outcomes for trials in hemodialysis: An international Delphi survey. *American Journal of Kidney Diseases*, 70(4), 464–475.

Gerteis, M., Edgman-Levitan, S., Daley, J., & Delbanco, T. (1993) *Through the Patient's Eyes: Understanding and Promoting Patient-Centered Care*. San Francisco, CA: Jossey-Bass.

Jain, A. K., Blake, P., Cordy, P. & Garg, A. X. (2012). Global trends in rates of peritoneal dialysis. *Journal of the American Society of Nephrology*, 23(3), 533–544.

Japanese NPO of Support for Patients with Kidney Diseases. (2019). *The Report of the Questionnaire Survey 2019*. Retrieved 12 September 2020, from https://www.kidney-directions.ne.jp/wp-content/themes/kidney-web/pdf/report/report_result_2019.pdf. (Japanese)

Japanese Society for Dialysis Therapy. (2019). 2018 Annual Dialysis Data Report, JSDT Renal Data Registry. *Nihon Toseki Igakkai Zassi*, 52(12), 679–754. Retrieved 18 July 2020, from https://docs.jsdt.or.jp/overview/file/2018/pdf/2018all.pdf.

Joseph-Williams, N., Lloyd, A., Edwards, A., Stobbart, L., Tomson, D., Macphail, S., … Thomson, R. (2017). Implementing shared decision making in the NHS: Lessons from the MAGIC programme. *BMJ*, 357, j1744.

Manera, K. E., Tong, A., Craig, J. C., Shen, J., Jesudason, S., Cho, Y., ... Johnson, D. W. (2019). An international Delphi survey helped develop consensus-based core outcome domains for trials in peritoneal dialysis. *Kidney International*, 96(3), 699–710.

Morton, R. L., Tong, A., Howard, K., Snelling, P., & Webster, A. C. (2010). The views of patients and carers in treatment decision making for chronic kidney disease: Systematic review and thematic synthesis of qualitative studies. *BMJ*, 340, c112.

Standardized Outcomes in Nephrology-Peritoneal Dialysis (SONG-PD) Workshop Investigators. (2020). Establishing a core outcome set for peritoneal dialysis: Report of the SONG-PD (Standardized Outcomes in Nephrology-Peritoneal Dialysis) consensus workshop. *American Journal of Kidney Diseases*, 75(3), 404–412.

The Joint Commission. (2020). *Speak Up Campaigns*. Retrieved 18 July 2020, from https://www.jointcommission.org/resources/for-consumers/speak-up-campaigns/.

The Royal College of Radiologists. (2016). *Standards for the Communication of Radiological Reports and Fail-safe Alert Notification*. London, The Royal College of Radiologists. Retrieved July 18 2020, from https://www.rcr.ac.uk/system/files/publication/field_publication_files/bfcr164_failsafe.pdf.

World Health Organization. (2007). *Patient Identification*. Patient Safety Solutions, volume 1, solution 2. Retrieved 18 July 2020, from https://www.who.int/patientsafety/solutions/patientsafety/PS-Solution2.pdf?ua=1.

15 'Muddling Through' Care Transitions

The Role of Patients and Their Families

Jane K. O'Hara, Ruth Baxter and Jenni Murray

CONTENTS

BACKGROUND

Transitions of care from hospital to home are risky. Shorter lengths of hospital stay (NHS Digital, 2016) and increased care delivery within community settings (NHS England, 2014) mean that patients often go home with ongoing treatment needs at a time when responsibilities for, and involvement in, their care is changing. Transitions of care are also complex. They are not neatly bounded within a single health care system but instead span multiple interacting systems that cross-professional, service, and organisational boundaries. Each system is organic in that it operates to its own priorities, rules, processes and procedures (Wears & Hunte, 2014). What constitutes 'safe' patient care varies by system and thus influences the actions that are taken to ensure safety. Together, these systems are only loosely coherent (Wears & Hunte, 2014) – they were not intentionally designed to support safe transitions.

Due to this complexity, high levels of performance variability and interdependence exist within and between the transitional care activities that are conducted across systems. Outcomes are therefore emergent but the adaptations of actors within each system ensure that, most of the time, transitional care 'goes right' – people continue their recovery and/or receive appropriate and safe care at home. The ability to ensure safe care is even more remarkable when considering transitions for older people. Variability is even greater within this patient population as people tend to have more complex health and social care needs (e.g., multiple comorbidities) and are more vulnerable to the deleterious effects of hospital care such as deconditioning (Boyd et al., 2008) and post-hospital syndrome (Krumholz, 2013).

Most outcomes for transitional care currently focus on negative events (e.g., readmissions, delayed transfers of care). Data on these outcomes indicate that there is scope to improve the safety and quality of transitions. For example, readmission rates have increased over time (Healthwatch England, 2017; NHS Digital, 2019); one in five patients report adverse events such as medication errors (Forster, Murff, Peterson, Gandhi, & Bates, 2003); and, patients and families often report negative experiences during the transitional period (Dossa, Bokhour & Hoenig, 2012; Georgiadis & Corrigan, 2017). Around 30% of readmissions (Auerbach et al., 2016; Blunt, Bardsley, Grove & Clarke, 2015) and two-thirds of adverse events are thought to be avoidable (Forster et al., 2003). As such, improving the safety and quality of transitional care is a priority for national and global health care systems.

This chapter begins by framing transitional care within the context of incrementalism. Using data from our own research, we discuss the safety gaps that arise as a result of incrementally designed systems and outline how health care professionals, patients, and families maintain safety during this period. We highlight the importance of combining these different perspectives and then describe how it may be possible to intervene by systematically supporting patients and families to bolster resilience during transitions of care.

'THE SCIENCE OF MUDDLING THROUGH' – WHAT CAN THIS ADD TO OUR UNDERSTANDING OF TRANSITIONAL CARE?

Incrementalism, or 'muddling through', has been explored in detail in an earlier chapter of this text, and we don't wish to duplicate this discussion. However, transitional care arguably represents an almost perfect exemplar of the role of incrementalism in amplifying variability. We contend that it is often only the movement *across* incrementally designed and developed services that can illuminate many of the safety issues that patients face *within* these separate health and social care services.

Lindblom (1959) argues that there are two main approaches to designing policy that shape how organisations meet their expressed functions: the 'root method' and the 'branch method'. In the 'root method', services are designed on the basis of a rational, comprehensive analysis where the ultimate ends are identified for the service, before the means to achieve those ends. The 'best' policies are those that maximise the range of values considered within the analysis. Within the context of incrementalism, we refer to 'values' as factors to be considered within an analysis, that are optimised through the design of the system or service.

Now, even the most naïve observer of health services would be hard pushed to argue that current health care systems have been designed using this method, if the value to be optimised was patient safety. It is clear that health services globally have been designed, like most services shaped by government policy, through 'successive incremental comparisons', or the 'branch method'. In this method, the analysis is based upon a more limited selection of values, and alternative possibilities, and often predicated on that oft-repeated idiom – 'start where you are'. While incrementalism, as it became known, has come to represent the cornerstone of public administration (Lindblom, 1979), it does present a number of significant problems with respect to patient safety – and in particular, the safety of transitional care – which we will explore in turn.

SUCCESSIVE LIMITED COMPARISONS LIMIT THE VALUES TO BE OPTIMISED

Designing services cannot be achieved by undertaking an exhaustive analysis of every possible value, and attempting to optimise all these values. Put simply, services are designed for a particular purpose – a means to a particular end – and to optimise a select number of pressures or directives. In acute care, some of the values to be optimised in designing and redeveloping services reflect quality, safety and efficiency within the boundaries of the hospital – *getting* people well and out of hospital as quickly as possible. These values might be very different from those used to design health care services for patients and the public within the community, which may reflect the need for *keeping* people well and out of hospital. This difference in the values around which the services are optimised may inadvertently amplify, or indeed cause, safety problems as patients move through the various systems and settings they encounter during transitions of care.

SAME VALUES, DIFFERENT INTERPRETATION?

Even where services may have the same espoused values – for example, 'delivering safe, quality care' – they may be realised in very different ways, with these differences likely to cause problems for patients and their families receiving care across different settings. Indeed, staff seeking to minimise safety risks *within* hospital might achieve these values in ways that actually conflict with the ways in which that same value is achieved *outside* of hospital. An example of this is in the almost universal falls reduction targets in acute care, which, while laudable, can have the unintended consequence of increasing the likelihood of falling once out of hospital, through physical deconditioning.

Evaluating Success Is Not 'Value-Neutral'

Incrementally designed services, based on a limited set of values, and meeting certain pre-specified objectives, cannot be argued to be judged neutrally on their 'success'. Performance feedback is by definition information sought by organisations to measure the meeting of pre-specified performance objectives. Put simply, if a service is designed to improve patient flow, improvements in patient flow will result in a positive judgement of the service if other values are not also measured, e.g., readmissions or patient experience. This can result in different services ostensibly attempting to optimise the same overarching value, in very different, and sometimes conflicting ways.

Incrementalism Shapes Behaviour within Services

While services might be optimised to achieve a certain set of limited values, individuals working within these services will have their own values, pressures and constraints. However, individual action is not independent of context, and incrementalism is very likely to shape behaviour. Diane Vaughan in her exploration of the Challenger spaceship disaster described an important phenomenon linked to incrementalism – the normalisation of deviance (Vaughan, 1996). She argued that activity within organisations is socially organised and systematically produced, and results in behaviour and decisions that can often be regarded as deviant to an outside observer, or after the fact. An example of this within transitional care might be the lack of attention to the discharge letter sent to primary care staff. While most lay people might consider this a crucial part of a successful transition home, this is an activity with such little value in hospitals that it is often given to the most junior medical staff, who have often never even met the patient. This task allocation might appear deviant to those outside the acute hospital environment, but completely congruent to those working within the values and prescribed norms of a service positioning patient flow as a more pressing concern.

In the next sections, we will explore and explicate these issues in more detail, using data from our work on transitional care, and in particular, how patients, families and staff can contribute to the resilience of the wider health service 'system', and mitigate some of the problems arising from incrementally designed health services.

MUDDLING THROUGH TRANSITION – THE STAFF PERSPECTIVE

Transitional care is delivered by various multidisciplinary health care professionals who work within and across teams, services, and organisational boundaries. To describe staff perspectives of how incrementalism impacts the safety of transitional care, we draw upon data that were collected as part of a study to explore how high performing health care teams deliver safe transitions to older people (Baxter et al., 2018, 2020). In brief, routine data were used to identify four hospital specialties and six general practices that displayed exceptionally low or reducing readmission rates over time. A total of 157 multidisciplinary health care professionals were recruited to participate in focus groups ($n = 21$) or one- or two-person interviews ($n = 12$). On hospital wards, meetings relating to discharge (e.g., multidisciplinary team meetings) were also observed. Participating staff included doctors, nurses, health care assistants, allied health professionals, discharge coordinators, and administrators who worked on wards within the hospital specialties and in the general practice teams. Community matrons, district nurses, and specialist nurses were also recruited from the community teams that worked into or with the high performing teams.

Although these data were not specifically collected to explore incrementalism, they highlight challenges with service design that staff have to navigate to deliver safe transitional care. Broadly, incremental changes to systems, processes, teams and services have culminated in 'transitions' of care being almost universally viewed as 'discharge' from hospital. Aligned to the four problems outlined in the section "'The science of muddling through" – what can this add to our understanding of transitional care?' we describe below how this may amplify safety issues during transitions, and how staff 'muddle through' to try and overcome them. In doing this, we hope to illuminate some of the resilient properties of the wider transitional care pathway.

First, teams, services, organisations and health care settings prioritise different values in the pursuit of delivering safe, effective, and efficient transitional care. With increasing demand for hospital beds (e.g., Ewbank, Thompson, McKenna & Anandaciva, 2020), a key value in secondary care is to get patients medically fit and ready for discharge as quickly as possible – i.e., to maintain patient flow through hospitals. Improved patient flow helps minimise patient risk (e.g., deconditioning, hospital-acquired infections), it aligns with patient and family preferences to be at home, and it helps alleviate organisational pressures (e.g., bed availability). Although each patient discharge represents an 'achievement' of this value, staff prioritise their attention towards existing and new patient admissions and, as such, have very little if no involvement in post-discharge care. Compounding this, primary and community care settings value keeping people well and out of hospital. Many patients require minimal or no post-discharge follow up (e.g., tests or monitoring) and so care is prioritised to those at risk of becoming unwell and to preventing hospital admissions in the first place. Recognising the 'safety gaps' that this creates during transitions of care, secondary care staff will push back against organisational hierarchies to discharge patients quickly while primary and community care staff will identify and prioritise patients who are vulnerable post-discharge or who have complex care needs, for example, by contributing to care pre-discharge or actively receiving patients at home.

Second, shared values were enacted differently across settings. Safe transitional care was almost universally perceived to be enhanced by having a holistic understanding of patient needs (i.e., wider psycho-social circumstances rather than just the medical situation) and through the involvement of patients and families. In secondary care, having a holistic understanding helped staff identify and mitigate transitional care risks, and patient and family involvement was predominantly characterised by gathering contextual information and collateral accounts to create safe discharge plans (e.g., information about the home environment or wider caring responsibilities). Some types of ward (e.g., complex discharge wards) felt they did this more effectively than others (e.g., admission or base wards), predominantly because they had time to get to know patients and uncover critical information. In general practice and community care settings staff were generally considered to have an even better understanding of patients' holistic needs as they provided care over, often lengthy, periods of time. This enabled them to tailor care to individuals, for example by referring patients to a broader range of health, social and voluntary sector services that would address their wider needs, rather than just those that were associated with the hospital admission. Furthermore, patient and family involvement was predominantly centred on education and encouraging self-management of their condition. This was at odds to secondary care settings where, in general, patients had limited 'responsibility' for their own care (e.g., medicines were dispensed by ward staff). At times, this disparity created unrealistic patient and/or family expectations regarding the care they could (or couldn't) expect to receive. Understanding the roles and constraints of colleagues in different health care settings helped staff set appropriate patient and family expectations.

Third, the prioritisation of transitional care measures differed across settings. In secondary care, measures and tools often aligned to improving patient flow. Meetings or dedicated clinical teams (e.g., complex discharge teams) were convened to try and reduce delayed transfers of care (when patients are considered ready for discharge but still occupy a hospital bed), and initiatives such as the SAFER Patient Flow Bundle and Red2Green days (NHS Improvement, 2020) were used to reduce delays within a patient's journey. In contrast, primary and community care settings used multidisciplinary team meetings (e.g., Gold Standard Framework meetings) as a forum for identifying patients who may be struggling or vulnerable to a hospital admission and reviewed data relating to out of hours health service contacts and admissions. Interestingly, regardless of setting, frontline staff held little value for emergency hospital readmission data which are used to measure the quality of transitional care nationally. Readmissions were predominantly considered to be unavoidable, and those that were potentially avoidable were rarely perceived to occur as a result of their own team's actions.

Fourth, values appeared to impact individual behaviour, particularly when handing over responsibility for patient care from one professional or team to another. In hospitals, the priority to get people medically fit meant that discharge letters and referrals were often written hurriedly, by junior doctors who may not have met or cared for the patient. Furthermore, hospital staff had limited or no role in supporting post-discharge care. As a result, primary and community care staff (who lacked capacity to be involved in patient care during a hospital admission) sometimes felt ill-equipped to take on responsibility for patient care post-discharge. The high performing health care teams took steps to try and minimise the impact the gap in responsibility had on safety. Junior doctors were trained to improve the quality of discharge letters and, when patient care was particularly complex, additional letters and/or verbal handovers were given. Primary and community care staff chased late, unclear, or inaccurate information in discharge letters/referrals via hospital teams, other health care professionals or through the patients and families themselves. In addition, infrastructure changes were implemented to try and improve the effectiveness, efficiency and safety of transitional care. However, these sometimes had unintended consequences. For example, centralised community nursing referral hubs were perceived to streamline referral processes, but they also made it more difficult to refer to or have discussions with specific individual staff members who would be caring for patients post-discharge. These systems could also create a false sense of security – and stymie the enactment of other 'resilient behaviours' – whereby care was assumed to be in place once the referral had been made. Similarly, electronic patient records and discharge letters provided primary and community care staff with more detailed or timely patient information, but they were not considered an adequate substitute for discussion between members of different health care teams – formal mechanisms for which were rarely available.

The next section will now juxtapose the problems experienced by staff, and the resilient behaviours or infrastructure props put in place to mitigate these, with the perspective of older patients and their families experiencing a transition from hospital to home.

BEING MUDDLED THROUGH TRANSITION – THE PATIENTS' PERSPECTIVE

Patients experience the various and cumulative consequences of incrementalism not within different parts of the system but within the context of their own journey between hospital and home. While patients often have a sense that demand for care will create a pressure to 'unblock' beds, they may not be privy to the values underpinning services and systems that shape staff behaviour. Nor will they necessarily understand the ways in which risks for them are exacerbated by different interpretations of the same values across different parts of the system. Patients therefore only know what they experience, largely without knowing exactly how that has come about. This section describes how older patients and their families experience transitions, drawing on where and how the problems presented by incrementalism impact on their own behaviours and safety. In describing this perspective, we draw upon data from a longitudinal focussed ethnography of the involvement and experience of 32 older patients (and 15 carers) during their from hospital stay to three months post-discharge (Hardicre et al., 2017, 2020).

PATIENTS' RESPONSIBILITIES IN HOSPITAL – A QUADRUPLE-EDGED SWORD

The quadruple-edged sword (if one existed) for patients is that on entry to the hospital, responsibility for care is both taken over *by* and handed over *to* the system, but that the discharge (or lead up to it) is not marked by deliberate and overt preparatory signals that responsibility for care will be handed back *to* and taken up *by* the patient. This creates a 'perfect storm' for patients, which only becomes fully apparent after discharge. As described previously, within hospitals 'safety values' are largely manifested in the pressure to maintain patient flow. A direct consequence of this is that in striving to 'get care done', care delivery often happens behind the scenes and is therefore invisible to patients. This is compounded by reduced staff-to-patient interaction, which further diminishes the opportunities to communicate vital information and therefore learning that may support patients to resume responsibility for their care once home. Interestingly, a value that is presented almost ubiquitously across hospitals is one of patient-centred care, patient 'empowerment' and involvement and it is here that we see how different values are expressed. The expression of the value of patient safety as patient flow, takes precedence over patient empowerment and involvement. Specific examples of how these processes impact on the patient are detailed below.

While in hospital many older patients will adopt a passive role, accepting care and organisational rules as they are presented to them (Murray, Hardicre, Birks, O'Hara & Lawton, 2019). Fear and acute ill-health will naturally compel many patients to place themselves wholly in the hands of professionals whose job it is to help them get better. Patients seem implicitly aware that being a 'good' patient means abiding by the 'rules' and not placing further burden on already busy staff. Many patients will be happy to let nursing care be 'done for' them including washing, dressing, feeding, and toileting. Minimising movement reduces the risks from falling and therefore supports patient flow. However, this can result in patients losing the skills and confidence required to complete these activities for themselves post-discharge, as well as physical deconditioning increasing the likelihood of falling once home. In an effort to balance safety risks across transitions, some wards will engage in campaigns such as 'End PJ Paralysis' (#EndPJparalysis, 2020), which promotes ward-based activities to help minimise physical deconditioning in hospital. Where these campaigns or similar approaches are absent or poorly implemented, patients who want to retain as much independence as possible may need to actively work against hospital processes, for example by mobilising around the ward despite being told not to. This requires extensive capacity and capability. However, patients who achieve this or who are supported to achieve this appear to be able to resume active involvement in their own care more easily at home.

SELF-MEDICATION IN HOSPITAL – WHOSE RISK IS IT ANYWAY?

Management of medicines in hospital is another example of safety values being operationalised in a way that causes problems for patients once home. On admission, patients' medicines are taken from them. Unbeknownst to patients, this is often not a recognised hospital policy, but the withdrawal of self-medication occurs as the expressed value of *safety within hospital* takes precedence. Clinical administration of medicines starts with decanting from labelled packets into cups, invariably without any patient involvement. This process creates an efficient mechanism whereby medicines can be dispensed across the ward to patients in rapid succession, and the risk of medication error is minimised. However, this creates problems for patients.

In hospital, we observed that patients are often not encouraged to ask questions during routine medication rounds or afforded the opportunity to practice taking medications. This can have the effect of reducing the self-efficacy for managing their medications. Further, because medicines are often altered in hospital due to changes in diagnosis or treatment, patients may fail to understand why they are on certain medicines or their potential side-effects. This lack of understanding risks both non-adherence as well as problems escalating when experiencing side effects or checking for prescription or administration errors.

THE SURPRISE OF DISCHARGE

The often held passive state that patients occupy, and in some ways the system relies on, continues throughout the patient stay. The invisible activities designed to optimise flow often brings about a sudden and surprising discharge announcement to unprepared patients. Critically, two key factors work together to lull patients into believing that a passive state of involvement can continue. Firstly, despite being declared medically fit or optimised for discharge, older patients can still feel unwell and therefore still feel the need for care and attention. Secondly, the discharge letter might refer to post-discharge care, or provide some reassurance that the 'receiving' health care community will know they are going home. This can create expectations for patients and families that they will be 'actively received' by primary or community care staff once home. However, as mentioned above, many primary and community care services will, despite an aspiration to offer care that is holistic, only be able to 'actively receive' patients who have specific, or complex medical needs, with the assumption that the majority will resume active self-care. With limited contact from clinical staff during this transitional period, patients may remain passive recipients of care, waiting for appointments that may not materialise, as unbeknownst to them, this is not a usual procedure for most patients. Unsurprisingly therefore, after discharge, patients will often feel that they have been abandoned through a lack of 'active receipt' by primary and community care services.

THE RESILIENCE OF PATIENTS AND FAMILIES

Despite the often experienced inadequacies of the discharge, and the lack of 'active receipt', patients and families do undertake activity that supports their care, and thus the resilience of the transitional care 'system'. For example, following discharge, some patients will, unprompted, approach their primary care doctor. When patients and families have good existing relationships with primary care staff, patients will sometimes take their discharge letters and old medication boxes to ensure they get the correct or new prescription. Additionally, patients and families may seek additional sources of information for help, such as internet searching or asking relatives and friends.

A TRANSITIONAL MUDDLE – COMBINING THESE PERSPECTIVES

In the preceding sections, we have presented examples from our studies on transitional care that illustrate some of the issues for delivering quality and safe care, across health care settings caused, or exacerbated by, incrementalism. These findings in and of themselves are perhaps not especially novel within the context of the extant empirical literature (e.g., Baillie et al., 2014; Kable, Chenoweth, Pond & Hullick, 2015; Waring, Bishop & Marshall, 2016). However, our work has attempted to take these findings one step further – to combine the perspectives of patients and families alongside those of health care staff, to create a novel understanding of the transitional care 'problem'.

Over the past few years, there has been an increasing recognition of the role of patients and families as contributors to the resilience of health care systems

(O'Hara, Aase, et al., 2019; O'Hara, Canfield, et al., 2019; Sujan, Furniss, Anderson, Braithwaite, & Hollnagel, 2019; Bergerød, Gilje, Braut, & Wiig, 2018; Fylan, Armitage, Naylor, & Blenkinsopp, 2018; Flyan, et al., 2019; Furniss, Barber, Lyons, Eliasson & Blandford, 2014; Schubert, Wears, Holden, & Hunte, 2015; Wiig et al., 2019). Patients and families may both introduce variability in systems (e.g., take medications, or not), as well undertake functional activity that effectively 'dampens' variability, thus contributing to resilience (e.g., chasing general practiioner appointments, question errors in prescriptions). For example, patients, their families and carers, can act as 'knowledge brokers', effectively carrying important information about their history, treatment and care around the health care system, and reducing the problems arising from safety gaps created by service infrastructure (O'Hara, Aase, et al., 2019). Patients and families may also 'step in' when systems fail, or are suboptimal, for example, undertaking their own medicines reconciliation following discharge on occasions where this has been omitted (Fylan et al., 2018; Furniss et al., 2014).

This particular framing of involvement by patients and families has been recently described as 'scaffolding our systems' (O'Hara, Aase et al., 2019) and 'co-creating resilience' (O'Hara, Canfield, et al., 2019). The key message from this framing is that a failure to recognise the activity undertaken by patients and families, as well as the variability (both 'wanted' and 'unwanted') that it introduces, risks incorrect assessments of the resilience of health care systems. In effect, not recognising the contribution of patients and families to system performance and outcomes could be regarded as an extension of 'Work-as-Imagined'.

To combine the perspectives of these different stakeholders, we undertook a functional resonance analysis using qualitative data from the two studies described in the preceding sections (Baxter et al., in press; Hardicre et al., 2020). This analysis has been described in detail within a previous publication (O'Hara, Baxter, & Hardicre, 2020). The functional resonance analysis method (FRAM) was chosen as a means of making sense of the transitional care system through the juxtaposition and combination of multiple stakeholders' perspectives of the same phenomenon. While the FRAM has been used previously as a means of combining multiple perspectives on a particular 'system' (e.g., Clay-Williams, Hounsgaard, & Hollnagel, 2015), this was the first published attempt to combine the perspectives of both the users, and providers of care, within one model. In creating our model, we sought to visually represent the functional activity undertaken within the system spanning admission of a patient into a hospital base ward, through to returning home, agnostic to whom – patients, families or health care staff – were undertaking the activity. Such an approach ultimately resulted in a new 'take' in an already crowded research field.

Figure 15.1 is a simplified version of our resultant FRAM model of transitional care, combining the perspectives of patients, families, carers and staff. Our modelling of the transitional care 'system' in this way led to a number of key conclusions about the nature of, and responsibility for, functional activity undertaken by patients and families following discharge home. We identified four key functions (activities) that following discharge became the responsibility of patients and families, that had previously been clinically managed or supported while in hospital. These functions are listed in Table 15.1.

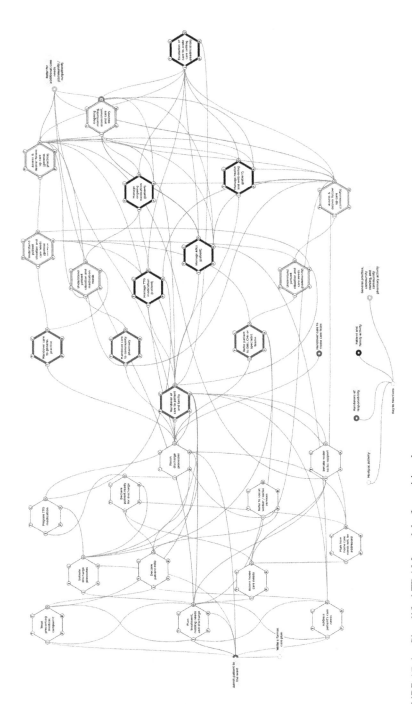

FIGURE 15.1   Simplified FRAM model of transitional care
(reproduced with permission; O'Hara et al., 2020)

TABLE 15.1

Functions undertaken by patient and families during transitional care

Title of Function (Activity)	Function
Activities of daily living (ADLs)	Patients and families have to resume and support activities often previously undertaken by clinical staff while in hospital, including mobilising, self-care and preparing meals.
Managing medication	Patients and families have to navigate the 'structural safety gap' that exists between hospital administered medications provided at discharge ('to-take-home' medications), and those prescribed by primary care and administered through community pharmacies. Further, patients and families have to undertake management of medication, and self-medicate as directed by the clinical staff.
Maintaining health and well-being	Patients and families have to manage the process of recovery following their hospital admission. This recovery is often not linear, and may involve monitoring of conditions, attending appointments, and escalating care when required.
Appropriately escalating care	Patients and families have to know when and where to escalate care. This is arguably a clinical decision that patients and families have to make routinely when they are at home. However, following an admission to hospital, decisions to escalate are particularly important and problematic for older patients and their families.

Through our FRAM analysis, we were able to identify a series of interdependencies between the four functional activities undertaken by patients and families at home, and the activities within hospital undertaken largely by clinical staff. As described in the preceding sections, through the design of health services in ways that can cause conflicting interpretations of 'safety', patients experience a sharp withdrawal of autonomy on admission to hospital, only to experience a sharp 'handing' back of this autonomy at discharge. Given that the functional activity undertaken by patients and families following discharge is largely, we argue, activity that was previously undertaken or supervised by clinical staff, we conceive this to be a 'handover to the patient' of the management of their health and care (O'Hara et al., 2020). When conceptualised like this, the way in which this handover is performed by services, and the credence given to this activity, is perhaps surprising. Our FRAM of transitional care supports the notion that what happens to patients and families in hospital, over and above their clinical condition and treatment, impacts directly on their ability to cope at home, their safety and the likelihood of readmission (O'Hara et al., 2020). Due to this interdependency between what happens in hospital and outcomes post-discharge, we conclude that patients and families may be better supported *within hospital* to achieve more successful 'outcomes' after returning home.

CAN WE SYSTEMATICALLY SUPPORT PATIENTS AND FAMILIES TO IMPROVE THE RESILIENCE OF TRANSITIONAL CARE?

We have argued that incrementalism as a basis for service design causes some particular issues for staff running these services, as well impacting on the experiences and outcomes for patients and families traversing these services. Our health care 'system' in fact represents the endpoint of millions of incrementally-made policy decisions, and even more decisions are made every day by staff and patients trying to optimise care within the framework of different (sometimes opposing) pressures, objectives and values. We contend that only through understanding the transitional care 'system' as experienced by multiple stakeholders – *including patients and families* – can we really understand how these incrementally designed services create structural 'safety gaps' for patients (O'Hara et al., 2018).

Our work, and that of other authors, has demonstrated that in addition to the resilient behaviours of health care staff, patients and families undertake activity that confers resilience to the transitional care 'system' (Fylan et al., 2018; Furniss et al., 2014). They 'step in' and mitigate the potential negative consequences where care is suboptimal, or the system fails, for example, when a referral is missed or medication is not prescribed. Therefore, one way to reduce the impact of our imperfect, incrementally designed services, and the structural 'safety gaps' these result in, might be to systematically support patients and families – in effect, create a 'scaffold' – to undertake these resilience activities when care falls short of what is needed to create safe outcomes.

There are some examples of interventions that recognise the imperfections in our health care systems, and the safety gaps that are created through incrementalism. For example, in the UK, we have seen improvement initiatives such as 'End PJ Paralysis' (#EndPJparalysis, 2020) which aims to reduce the physical deconditioning associated with hospital. Further, the 'Red Bag' scheme (NHS England, 2018) aims to reduce the safety gaps created when a care home resident is admitted to hospital, enabling a timely sharing of important information such as current medications and patient history. However, most of these interventions fail to reduce some of the most problematic issues for patients caused by incrementalism – the complex and often opaque network of health care professionals across settings, and the multiplicity and limitations of different accountable care organisations and clinical responsibilities. Put simply, patients and families often cannot 'step in' when care fails because they lack the understanding, competence or physical capability to do so.

THE 'YOUR CARE NEEDS YOU' INTERVENTION

Our work on transitional care has led to the development of the 'Your Care Needs You' intervention (YQSR, 2020). This intervention aims to support patients in hospital to retain the capacities – physical and psychological – required to function safely when they get home, as well as provide opportunities to understand how their hospital admission will impact upon them following discharge. In keeping with the guidance for the development of complex interventions (e.g., O'Cathain et al., 2019), in addition to drawing on existing theory to underpin an intervention, it is also important to develop a programme specific theory of change that explicates how and why the specific components of an intervention may effect change in the desired outcomes. This is important, as 'articulating programme theory at the start of the development process can help to communicate to funding agencies and stakeholders how the intervention will work' (O'Cathain et al., 2019, p. 7). Therefore, we took the learning from our FRAM analysis, and translated it into a programme theory for the

YCNY intervention, which we visualised as a logic model (see Figure 15.2). Based upon the four functional activities undertaken by patients and families at home (see previous section and Table 15.1), the YCNY intervention supports patients to 'know more' and 'do more' while they are in hospital. The basic premise of this intervention is to encourage patients to 'practise for being at home' during their hospital stay. This practising supports retention of current competence and capacity, as well as development of any new knowledge and skills required to take on 'responsibility' for the four key patient-led activities post-discharge, thereby enhancing system resilience.

To enable this, the intervention (in its current form) comprises both patient- and staff-facing components. The patient-facing components include a YCNY booklet, a short film and instructions for going home. The booklet provides information about the importance of patients preparing for home while still in hospital. It highlights things that patients and families should know, supports them to ask questions of staff, and suggests how they could gain or retain the skills and confidence required for them to manage their care safely post-discharge – for example, by mobilising and practising taking medications. The film, to be shown to patients early in their hospital admission, emphasises the importance of practising to manage at home. The 'Patient Instructions for Home' document supports the handover of responsibility to patients occurring at discharge. It provides information on what to expect and how to seek help if needed – effectively supporting the systematic 'reaching in' by patients and families when care falls short of what is needed.

Despite these intervention components, older patients and their families may still struggle to enact involvement throughout their hospital stay (Murray et al., 2019). As such, the intervention also comprises a range of staff facing options that staff can develop and adapt to support patients in their efforts to know and do more. How staff

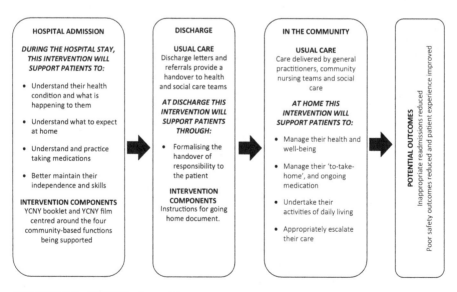

FIGURE 15.2   YCNY logic model
(adapted from O'Hara et al., 2020)

support and encourage patients to do this will vary by ward. This flexibility allows the YCNY intervention to tap into the resilience that staff, patients and families already demonstrate during transitions of care. It also aligns with recent literature that suggests interventions should be standardised according to their functional aims (in this case the four patient-facing post-discharge activities) rather than their form or components (e.g., Hawe, 2015; Hawe et al., 2004).

A feasibility trial has been undertaken (Baxter et al., 2020) which suggests that the YCNY intervention is feasible and acceptable for staff and patients. In 2020–2021, a 40-ward cluster randomised controlled trial is being undertaken across up to nine NHS Trusts in the North of England. This will establish the effectiveness of the YCNY intervention in improving the safety and experience of transitional care for older people, and thus reducing the likelihood of experiencing an emergency hospital readmission. In addition, we will be undertaking a process evaluation to explore the assumptions within our programme theory, to understand if patients and families can be systematically supported to 'step into' the safety gaps that arise as a result of incrementally designed transitional care 'system'.

CONCLUSION

In this chapter, we have explored the issues for transitional care caused, or exacerbated by, incrementalism. We have demonstrated that both providers and receivers of care act in ways that reduce these problems, and thus impact upon the resilience of the transitional care 'system'. We have argued that only through considering the multiplicity of perspectives from both receivers and providers of care, can we really understand how variability is introduced – or dampened – across transitional care.

From our analysis, we can say with some confidence that 'muddling through' transitional care safely not only relies on the resilient actions of health care professionals, but also patients and their families. However, can we systematically support patients and families to improve the resilience of transitional care? We don't have the answer to that question yet. There are certainly aspects of hospital admission – medication, mobility, and basic information about condition, treatment and care – that health services could improve to support patients and their families support themselves once they are home. For some patients, being able to practise in hospital those activities that they will resume responsibility for once home seems sensible, and indeed possible. However, such service redesign will not come without considerable challenges, particularly where patients do not want, or are not able to embrace responsibility for care, and where staff struggle to view patients as contributing positively to system resilience. Hopefully, through ongoing research and critical reflection, we can work out how, and if, these challenges can be overcome.

ACKNOWLEDGEMENTS

Data reported in this chapter is independent research funded by the National Institute for Health Research (NIHR) Programme Grants for Applied Health Research, Partners at Care Transitions (PACT): Improving patient experience and safety at transitions in care, RP-PG-1214-20017. Jane O'Hara is supported by the National Institute for Health Research Yorkshire and Humber Patient Safety Translational Research Centre (NIHR Yorkshire and Humber PSTRC). The views expressed in this publication are those of the authors and not necessarily those of the NIHR or the Department of Health and Social Care. The authors would like to thank the wider research team, in particular Rebecca Lawton, Rosie Shannon, Natasha Hardicre, Lesley Hughes and Laura Sheard.

REFERENCES

#EndPJParalysis (2020). Retrieved 12 June 2020, from https://endpjparalysis.org/

Auerbach, A. D., Kripalani, S., Vasilevskis, E. E., Sehgal, N., Lindenauer, P. K., Metlay, J. P., … Williams, M. V. (2016). Preventability and Causes of Readmissions in a National Cohort of General Medicine Patients. *JAMA Internal Medicine*, 176(4):484–493.

Baillie, L., Gallini, A., Corser, R., Elworthy, G., Scotcher, A., & Barrand, A. (2014). Care transitions for frail, older people from acute hospital wards within an integrated healthcare system in England: A qualitative case study. *International Journal of Integrated Care*, 14, e009.

Baxter, R., Murray, J., O'Hara, J. K., Hewitt, C., Richardson, G., Cockayne, S., … Lawton, R. (2020). Improving patient experience and safety at transitions of care through the Your Care Needs You (YCNY) intervention: A study protocol for a cluster randomised controlled feasibility trial. *Pilot and Feasibility Studies*. Retrieved from http://eprints.whiterose.ac.uk/164417/.

Baxter, R., O'Hara, J., Murray, J., Sheard, L., Cracknell, A., Foy, R., … Lawton, R. (2018). Partners at care transitions: Exploring healthcare professionals' perspectives of excellence at care transitions for older people. *BMJ Open*, 8(9), e022468.

Baxter, R., Shannon, R., Murray, J., O'Hara, J. K., Sheard, L., Cracknell, A., & Lawton, R. (2020). Delivering exceptionally safe transitions of care to older people: A qualitative study of multidisciplinary staff perspectives. *BMC Health Services Research*, 20, 780.

Bergerød, I.J., Gilje, B., Braut, G.S., & Wiig, S. (2018). Next-of-kin involvement in improving hospital cancer care quality and safety – A qualitative cross-case study as basis for theory development. *BMC Health Services Research*, 18(1), 324.

Blunt, I., Bardsley, M., Grove, A., & Clarke, A. (2015). Classifying emergency 30-day readmissions in England using routine hospital data 2004–2010: What is the scope for reduction? *Emergency Medicine Journal*, 32(1), 44–50.

Boyd, C. M., Landefeld, C. S., Counsell, S. R., Palmer, R. M., Fortinsky, R. H., Kresevic, D., … Covinsky, K. E. (2008). Recovery of activities of daily living in older adults after hospitalization for acute medical illness. *Journal of the American Geriatrics Society*, 56(12), 2171–2179.

Clay-Williams, R., Hounsgaard, J., & Hollnagel, E. (2015). Where the rubber meets the road: Using FRAM to align work-as-imagined with work-as-done when implementing clinical guidelines. *Implementation Science*, 10(1), 125.

Dossa, A., Bokhour, B., & Hoenig, H. (2012). Care transitions from the hospital to home for patients with mobility impairments: Patient and family caregiver experiences. *Rehabilitation Nursing*. 37, 277–285.

Ewbank, L., Thompson, J., McKenna, H., & Anandaciva, S. (2020). *NHS Hospital Bed Numbers: Past, Present, Future.* London, UK: The Kings Fund.

Forster, A. J., Murff, H. J., Peterson, J. F., Gandhi, T. K., & Bates, D. W. (2003). The incidence and severity of adverse events affecting patients after discharge from the hospital. *Annals of Internal Medicine*, 138(3), 161–167.

Furniss, D., Barber, N., Lyons, I., Eliasson, L., & Blandford, A. (2014). Unintentional non-adherence: Can a spoon full of resilience help the medicine go down? *BMJ Quality and Safety*, 23(2), 95–98.

Fylan, B., Armitage, G., Naylor, D., & Blenkinsopp, A. (2018). A qualitative study of patient involvement in medicines management after hospital discharge: An under-recognised source of systems resilience. *BMJ Quality and Safety*, 27(7), 539–546.

Fylan, B., Marques, I., Ismail, H., Breen, L., Gardner, P., Armitage, G., & Blenkinsopp, A. (2019). Gaps, traps, bridges and props: A mixed-methods study of resilience in the medicines management system for patients with heart failure at hospital discharge. *BMJ Open*, 9(2), e023440.

Georgiadis, A, & Corrigan, O. (2017). The experience of transitional care for non-medically complex older adults and their family caregivers. *Global Qualitative Nursing Research*, 4, 1–9.

Hardicre, N. K., Birks, Y., Murray, J., Sheard, L., Hughes, L., Heyhoe, J., … Lawton, R. (2017). Partners at Care Transitions (PACT) – Exploring older peoples' experiences of transitioning from hospital to home in the UK: Protocol for an observation and interview study of older people and their families to understand patient experience and involvement in care at transitions. *BMJ Open*, 7(11), e018054.

Hardicre, N. K., Shannon, R., Murray, J., Sheard, L., Birks, Y., Hughes, L., … Lawton, R. (2020). *'Involvement work': A qualitative study exploring how older people enact care involvement during transition from hospital to home*. Manuscript submitted for publication.

Hawe, P. (2015). Lessons from complex interventions to improve health. *Annual Review of Public Health*, 36, 307–323.

Hawe, P., Shiell, A., & Riley, T. (2004). Complex interventions: How "out of control" can a randomised controlled trial be? *British Medical Journal*, 328(7455), 1561–1563.

Healthwatch England. (2017). *What Do the Numbers Say About Emergency Readmissions to Hospital?*, Newcastle, UK: Healthwatch England.

Kable, A., Chenoweth, L., Pond, D., & Hullick, C. (2015). Health professional perspectives on systems failures in transitional care for patients with dementia and their carers: A qualitative descriptive study. *BMC Health Services Research*, 15(1), 567.

Krumholz, H. M. (2013). Post-Hospital Syndrome – An Acquired, Transient Condition of Generalized Risk. *New England Journal of Medicine*, 368(2), 100–102.

Lindblom, C. E. (1959). The science of "muddling through". *Public Administration Review*, 19(2), 79–88.

Lindblom, C. E. (1979). Still muddling, not yet through. *Public Administration Review*. 39(6), 517–526.

Murray, J., Hardicre, N., Birks, Y., O'Hara, J., & Lawton, R. (2019). How older people enact care involvement during transition from hospital to home: A systematic review and model. *Health Expectations*, 22(5), 883–893.

NHS Digital (2016). *Hospital Admitted Patient Care Activity 2015–16*. Leeds, UK: NHS Digital. Retrieved 10 June 2020, from https://files.digital.nhs.uk/publicationimport/pub22xxx/pub22378/hosp-epis-stat-admi-summ-rep-2015-16-rep.pdf.

NHS Digital (2019). *Emergency Readmissions Published for First Time in Five Years*. Leeds, UK: NHS Digital. Retrieved 30 September 2019, from https://digital.nhs.uk/news-and-events/latest-news/emergency-readmissions-published-for-first-time-in-five-years.

NHS England (2014). *Five Year Forward View*. London, UK: NHS. Retrieved 10 June 2020, from https://www.england.nhs.uk/wp-content/uploads/2014/10/5yfv-web.pdf.

NHS England (2018). *'Red bags' to be Rolled Out Across England's Care Homes Getting Patients Home from Hospital Quicker*. London, UK: NHS. Retrieved 3 September 2020, from https://www.england.nhs.uk/2018/06/red-bags-to-be-rolled-out-across-englands-care-homes-getting-patients-home-from-hospital-quicker/.

NHS Improvement (2020). *SAFER Patient Flow Bundle*. Retrieved 10 June 2020, from https://improvement.nhs.uk/resources/safer-patient-flow-bundle-implement/.

O'Cathain, A., Croot, L., Duncan, E., Rousseau, N., Sworn, K., Turner, K. M., ... Hoddinott, P. (2019). Guidance on how to develop complex interventions to improve health and healthcare. *BMJ Open*, 9(8), e029954.

O'Hara, J. K., Aase, K., & Waring, J. (2019). Scaffolding our systems? Patients and families 'reaching in' as a source of healthcare resilience. *BMJ Quality and Safety*, 28(1), 3–6.

O'Hara, J. K., Baxter, R., & Hardicre, N. (2020). 'Handing over to the patient': A FRAM analysis of transitional care combining multiple stakeholder perspectives. *Applied Ergonomics*. 85, 103060.

O'Hara, J. K., Canfield, C., & Aase, K. (2019). Patient and family perspectives in resilient healthcare studies: A question of morality or logic? *Safety Science*,120, 99–106.

Schubert, C.C., Wears, R.L., Holden, R.J., Hunte, G.S., (2015). Patients as a source of resilience. In R. Wears, E. Hollnagel, & J. Braithwaite (Eds.), *Resilient Health Care, Volume 2: The Resilience of Everyday Clinical Work* (pp. 207–224). Farnham, UK: Ashgate Publishing.

Sujan, M. A., Furniss, D., Anderson, J., Braithwaite, J., & Hollnagel, E. (2019). Resilient Health Care as the basis for teaching patient safety – A Safety-II critique of the World Health Organisation patient safety curriculum. *Safety Science*, 118, 15–21.

Vaughan, D. (1996). *The Challenger Launch Decision: Risky Technology, Culture, and Deviance at NASA*. Chicago, IL: University of Chicago Press.

Waring, J., Bishop, S., & Marshall, F. (2016). A qualitative study of professional and carer perceptions of the threats to safe hospital discharge for stroke and hip fracture patients in the English National Health Service. *BMC Health Services Research*, 16(1), 297

Wears, R. L., & Hunte, G. S. (2014). Seeing patient safety 'Like a State'. *Safety Science*, 67, 50–57.

Wiig, S., Schibevaag, L., Tvete Zachrisen, R., Hannisdal, E., Anderson, J.E., & Haraldseid-Driftland, C. (2019). Next of kin involvement in regulatory investigation of adverse events that caused patient death: A process evaluation (part II inspectors' perspective). *Journal of Patient Safety*. [Epublication ahead of print]. doi:10.1097/PTS.0000000000000634.

YQSR – The Yorkshire Quality and Safety Research Group (2020). *Your Care Needs You*. Retrieved 12 June 2020, from www.yqsr.org/ycny.

Part V

Closure

CLOSURE

We now conclude the sixth volume of the Resilient Health Care series. In this closing chapter, Braithwaite, Hollnagel and Hunte bring the book to a culmination, offering a synthesis of the work of the chapters, and in doing so, providing two key concluding messages: that resilient performance comprises purposive muddling and that the incremental concept describes the work of everyone in health care. Together these messages may aid how stakeholders, whether within or external to the systems of care, understand what happens around them. Providers or recipients, workers or commentators, researchers or the researched: all can benefit, we believe, from an appreciation of Lindblom's original outline of muddling and our contemporary assessment of the place of muddling in resilient performance (Figure 1)

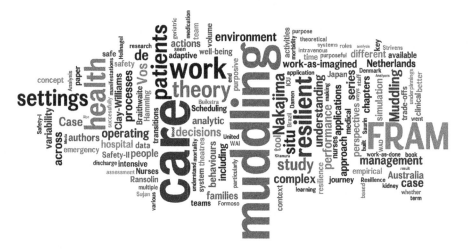

FIGURE 1   A word cloud of Part V. (Source: http://www.wordle.net/)

16 Conclusion

*Jeffrey Braithwaite, Erik Hollnagel and
Garth Hunte*

We started this sixth volume in the Resilient Health Care series by documenting how we asked the contributors to consider how clinicians, associated health workers, managers and policymakers proceed through the day, make decisions and do their work in adaptive and flexible ways – essentially, muddling through with purpose. We especially wanted to consider how decisions are reached and actions arise out of those decisions, whether about what to do next, what to do for a planned course of action, or what to do in the long run.

Whether for immediate, medium-term or long-term purposes, many people like to think of decisions and actions as the timely result of rational and conscious thought. But in practice decisions are made and actions emanate on the spot to fit the situation as it is seen and understood in the moment. This manner of coping with current constraints and exploiting opportunities has been described as muddling through by Charles E Lindblom in his now classic 1959 paper 'The science of "muddling through" and his follow-up paper 20 years later, "Still muddling, not yet through"' (Lindblom, 1959, 1979).

Although the term has struck a chord with many people over the years, and been supplemented by like-minded constructs with names such as incrementalism, gradualism, adaptive actions, taking 'baby-steps', degrees of manoeuvrability, and evolutionary rather than revolutionary approaches, few scholars have seriously and deeply grappled with the idea and its consequences for today's complex work environments. In particular, theories and empirical studies about muddling and the delivery of safe patient care have not been brought together in a book-length volume before.

***

Everywhere you look in health care there are muddling activities: people getting by, operating under less than perfect conditions and executing multi-faceted roles. Their activities are characterised by diffuse decision-making, efficiency-thoroughness trade-offs, improvisation and emergent, unplanned behaviours – as we have seen in the chapters which preceded this conclusion. Neither we nor the chapter writers have used 'muddling' as a pejorative term as some do ('everyone is making it up as they go along'), but as a descriptive and analytic term ('how are productive behaviours enacted in complex, ambiguous, deceptive, sometimes chaotic and always uncertain settings?'). The authors sought to understand how safe care is successfully delivered in such circumstances.

In order to better realise the potential for resilient health care across settings, the chapters accomplished several things. For example, they elucidated how muddling actions emerge, as we saw in the Patterson and Deutsch chapter on in situ simulation, in Takizawa, Mieda, Yokohama and Nakajima's study of blood transfusions, in Jackson's research on nurses accounting for Work-as-Imagined after playing her *Resilience Challenge* game, and in O'Hara, Baxter and Murray's work on the transitions of patients and families from hospital to home.

The authors were able to reflect on the manifestation of purposive muddling in real-world health settings as different as the hospital care of kidney patients in Japan (Kitamura and Nakajima); in Dutch Mortality and Morbidity case meetings (Hamming and de Vos); in Brazilian intensive care settings (Ransolin, Suarin and Formoso); in a geriatric ward environment (Buikstra, Clay-Williams and Strivens); in Japanese emergency medical teams (Nakamura, Nakajima, Nakajima and Abe); and in French operating suite ecosystems (Mahmoud, Sarkies, Clay-Williams, Saurin and Braithwaite).

We also saw deep, considered analysis of the explanatory power of the muddling concept via a series of Functional Resonance Analysis Method (FRAM) applications. Damen and de Vos's research from the Netherlands looked across multiple topics including preoperative anticoagulation management, radiology, postpartum haemorrhage, thrombosis prophylaxis and how triaging works in emergency settings. Meanwhile, 19,000 kilometres distant from Damen and de Vos in Europe, Buikstra, Clay-Williams and Strivens in Townsville, in Queensland Australia were examining the discharge processes for geriatric patients, also in inpatient settings. Sujan from the UK and Ransolin, Suarin and Formoso from Brazil were both interested in intensive care settings but from different angles; in Sujan's case, by focussing on intravenous medication ordering, and in the Ransolin et al. case, looking at the intersection of the built environment of the intensive care setting and its influence on patient safety and well-being.

Collectively, these applied descriptions of the variability of everyday performance reflected on how to dampen unwanted variability and how to amplify desirable variability. FRAM is a tool for identifying dynamic work patterns such as when people are creating room for manoeuvre, doing workarounds, and coping with things that have never happened before – all characteristic of purposive muddling behaviours in relevant settings.

This growing understanding of muddling in situ was based not only on the evidence provided by our multiple empirical chapters, but also conceptual work such as the big data proposals of de Vos and Hamming from the Netherlands. As always, the Resilient Health Care series aims to provide practical value to stakeholders who want to explore the potential of resilient health care and apply the ideas to their work.

***

By way of further distilling the work of the chapters we present Table 16.1. This helps draw out the salient points from the wide-ranging and more detailed contributions of each author.

Altogether this volume continues the quest of the Resilient Health Care series (Hollnagel, Braithwaite, & Wears 2013; Wears, Hollnagel, & Braithwaite, 2015; Braithwaite, Wears, & Hollnagel, 2017; Hollnagel, Braithwaite and Wears 2019 & Braithwaite, Hollnagel, & Hunte, 2019) to explicate real-world care. As authors and editors, we have prosecuted the case for the importance of recognising and understanding muddling actions, practices and activities in order to create resilient performance in health care. The point of *Muddling Through with Purpose* was to demonstrate how resilient health care principles can enable everyone – whether at the

TABLE 16.1

A summary of the book – authors, lessons, country, empirical stance and theoretical approach

Authors, Chapter	Selected Key Lessons	Country	Empirical Stance	Theoretical Approach
Part I: Openings				
Braithwaite, Hollnagel and Hunte Introduction: how we got to here	Prior volumes in the series focussed on resilience and everyday clinical work, Work-as-Imagined and Work-as-Done, research and theory on ways to deliver resilient health care and the context of complexity of social structures and different kinds of boundary-crossing actions. Now, we discuss resilient health care in the context of purposeful muddling and incrementalism.	Australia, Denmark, Canada	Historical background and context of Volumes 1–5	Introduction and conceptual overview
Hollnagel The necessity of muddling through	Since we can never know all the alternatives or distinguish between them, muddling is necessary – and needs to be understood as such.	Denmark	Examines the historical context for muddling; establishes the concept of muddling.	Sketches briefly some of the key theoretical underpinnings for muddling.
Part II: Case studies of muddling				
Mahmoud, Sarkies, Clay-Williams, Saurin and Braithwaite Managing complexity and manifestations of resilience in operating theatres: sensemaking and purposive muddling among Scheduling Nurses	Scheduling Nurses in operating theatres undertook complex work such as organising patient processes, juggling different perspectives and making complex decisions, navigating the gaps between Work-as-Imagined and Work-as-Done. Goals between surgeons and Scheduling Nurses frequently conflicted, but flexible and accommodating social structures helped deal with variability in workflow and performance.	France, Australia, Brazil	Case study of Scheduling Nurses in operating theatres.	Resilience theory meets Lean application.
Takizawa, Mieda, Yokohama and Nakajima Re-designing the blood transfusion procedure in operating theatres: aligning Work-as-Imagined and Work-as-Done.	Analyses the entanglement of paper based and digital systems in transitioning from a paper based to a barcoding system. The *genba* (Japanese for the actual workplace) was observed and a new system to ensure patients were kept safe was instituted.	Japan	Multidisciplinary team discussion: questionnaire surveys and a follow up educational visit.	Work-as-Imagined and Work-as-Done.

(continued)

Authors, Chapter	Selected Key Lessons	Country	Empirical Stance	Theoretical Approach
Nakamura, Nakajima, Nakajima and Abe Dynamic performance of emergency medical teams as seen in responses to unexpected clinical events	Emergency medical teams facing a mass casualty incident allocated roles as interim arrangements and then fine-tuned resources and roles, making fine adjustments when time was available. This proved to be an effective and resilient method.	Japan	Assessment of an emergency medical team under crisis conditions.	Resilience theory: Work-as-Imagined and Work-as-Done: likening the changing shape of the team to slime mould.
Hamming and de Vos From Mortality and Morbidity conference to Quality Assessment Meeting: step-by-step improving team resilience	A review of learning from what went right, not just what went wrong in Mortality and Morbidity conferences. Further refinements to the model over time should include the input of nursing staff and other disciplinary input including from anaesthesiologists and intensivists.	The Netherlands	Case study of Mortality and Morbidity meetings over time.	Quality improvement theory and learning from what goes right.
Jackson Images of Work-as-Imagined	Assessment of nurses' views of their work, capturing their perspectives of Work-as-Imagined and Work-as-Done. Work-as-Imagined for nurses include policies, and also aspects of culture and professional image.	Canada	Interviews ($N = 20$) with nurses.	Analysis of perspective on Work-as-Imagined.
Part III: Functional Resonance Analysis Method (FRAM) as a gateway into muddling with a purpose				
Damen and de Vos Experiences with FRAM in Dutch hospitals: muddling through with models	Discussion of various applications of FRAM including optimising processes, investigating incidents and developing and implementing guidelines and interventions. A synthesis is provided with suggestions about the ways to proceed with future FRAM applications, alongside a brief assessment of its strengths and challenges.	The Netherlands	FRAM as an analytic tool in situ, ranging across multiple case exemplars.	The underpinnings and manifestations of FRAM applications.

(continued)

Authors, Chapter	Selected Key Lessons	Country	Empirical Stance	Theoretical Approach
Buikstra, Clay-Williams and Strivens Modelling a typical patient journey through the Geriatric Evaluation and Management Ward to better understand discharge planning processes	An in-depth assessment of FRAM in a geriatric evaluation and management ward. Examines the need for trade-offs between thoroughness and efficiency, for example, and helps aid understanding of how clinicians muddle through to meet organisational and patient needs.	Australia	FRAM as an analytic tool in situ looking at the specific examples of muddling and the connection between inpatients and discharge processes.	FRAM theory and manifestations via a case approach.
Sujan Muddling through in the intensive care unit – a FRAM analysis of intravenous infusion management	FRAM as applied to intravenous medication management in an ICU, and its strengths and weaknesses are considered in particular regarding trade-offs in other activities. Discusses the tensions and contradictions in clinical work and the utility of FRAM in understanding this.	United Kingdom	FRAM as an analytic tool in situ to study specific medication management issues.	FRAM theory in relation particularly to trade-offs.
Ransolin, Saurin and Formoso Muddling through the built environment to preserve patient safety and well-being	Investigates the relationship between the built environment of an ICU and patient safety and well-being, mediated by human factors.	Brazil	FRAM as an analytic tool in situ to examine ICU performance.	Built environment theory, patient safety and well-being theory and FRAM theory.

Part IV: Muddling with application: in and around hospitals

Authors, Chapter	Selected Key Lessons	Country	Empirical Stance	Theoretical Approach
Patterson and Deutsch Simulation to surface adaptive capacity	A study of how in situ simulation can assist learning while minimising direct patient risks. The benefits of this mechanism include supporting individuals, clinical teams and broader systems of care.	United States of America	Analysis of in situ simulation across different applications including during Covid-19.	Theories of simulation particularly the direct application of simulation and its contribution to clarifying adaptive capacity.

(continued)

Authors, Chapter	Selected Key Lessons	Country	Empirical Stance	Theoretical Approach
de Vos and Hamming Towards Safety-II in hospital care using the available Safety-I environment: patient-level linkage of currently available hospital data	Looks at the benefits of conjoining Safety-II principles with Safety-I processes in systems, particularly in terms of available hospital data. Demonstrates how such analyses can reveal aspects of successful performance.	The Netherlands	Case study approach to using big data sets in a Safety-II frame.	Data management theories, Safety-I and Safety-II.
Kitamura and Nakajima Peer-to-peer information sharing for a high-quality, autonomous and efficient health care system	Patients as key human resources in the care process is much discussed and less researched than many would prefer: the patient journey of those with chronic kidney disease is analysed. Patients with chronic kidney disease in a peer-to-peer relationship can successfully help each other across time.	Japan	Case study approach and supporting the journey of peritoneal dialysis patients.	Patient journey theory; peer-to-peer information sharing.
O'Hara, Baxter and Murray 'Muddling through' care transitions – the role of patients and their families	Analyses the risky and complex episodes when patients transit from one part of health care to another. There are many and differing perspectives to be understood including those of the staff and the patients and their families. The end result is to reduce variability and risks in transitions.	United Kingdom	Case study of various transitions involving patients and their families.	Transitions theory; triangulated perspectives of staff, patients and families.
Part V: Closure				
Braithwaite, Hollnagel and Hunte Conclusion	Muddling is a useful concept to understand purposeful actions in resilient settings. The wide-ranging empirical and theoretical perspectives add depths of understanding to these phenomena.	Australia, Denmark, Canada	Critical synthesis of prior material.	Theoretical pluralities.

blunt end, the sharp end, or as an external stakeholder with an interest in seeing better health care for patients – to work more effectively towards safe, high-quality, inter-disciplinary care by gaining a deeper understanding of real-world improvisations that manifest in all care settings.

We hope that readers will see, as they digest the work of the chapter authors, that *Muddling Through with Purpose* has two key messages: first, in line with the over-arching goal of this contribution to the book series, we can now appreciate more clearly that resilient performance requires purposive muddling. Put differently, we might say that if resilience is the scaffolding of any successful system, muddling with purpose is the underpinning of action.

The second message is that it is helpful for all of us to be aware of our own pur-poseful muddling, as mirrored across the pages of the chapters in this book. The concept evocatively describes everyone's work, not just the subjects of our chapter writers, whether engaged in working as a policymaker, regulator or researcher, or leading, or managing, or practising clinically on the frontlines of care. We hope that this volume will help people be better informed, and become more adept at solving problems in dynamic settings – to function effectively and operate successfully among the multitude of complex ecosystems we call 'health care'.

REFERENCES

Braithwaite, J., Hollnagel, E., & Hunte, G. (Eds). (2019) *Resilient Health Care, Volume 5: Working Across Boundaries*. Boca Raton, FL: CRC Press.

Braithwaite, J., Wears, R. L., & Hollnagel, E. (Eds.). (2017). *Resilient Health Care, Volume 3: Reconciling Work-as-Imagined and Work-as-Done*. Boca Raton, Fl: CRC Press.

Hollnagel, E., Braithwaite, J., & Wears, R. (Eds.). (2013). *Resilient Health Care*. Farnham, Surrey: Ashgate Publishing.

Hollnagel, E., Braithwaite, J., & Wears, R. (Eds) (2019) *Resilient Health Care, Volume 4: Delivering Resilient Health Care*. Abingdon, UK: Routledge.

Lindblom, CE. (1959), The science of "muddling through". *Public Administration Review*, 19(2), 79–88.

Lindblom, CE. (1979), Still muddling, not yet through. *Public Administration Review*, 39(6), 517–526.

Wears, R., Hollnagel, E., & Braithwaite, J. (Eds.). (2015). *Resilient Health Care, Volume 2: The Resilience of Everyday Clinical Work*. Farnham, UK: Ashgate Publishing.

Index

Printed in the United States
by Baker & Taylor Publisher Services